THE CARED FOR

By

Craig Henry

For Carolyn

Contents

ACKNOWLEDGEMENTS

This book would not have been possible without all the incredible people that have taken care of me over the last year. Thank you to all the hospital staff who went above and beyond to look after me even when I was being a nuisance. To all the patients I met along the way you gave me so much and whenever you are now, you're in my heart. To my second family, the Melbourne's. Your unwavering kindness, love and support was more than I ever deserved. Kindest Peter, Sarah, Katy and Dulcie for carrying me through my darkest of days. You have lifted my spirits and given me the opportunity to live another day. I am so grateful for every card, text, hug, Facebook message, prayer and that junior doctor who gave me the nudge to write this book.

Finally, to my dearest Elizabeth for believing in me when I forgot how to and showing me that love truly can conquer all.

Merry Christmas

"Given your family history and the fact your leg feels swollen, I would suggest an urgent appointment at the Royal Marsden Hospital to get yourself checked out." Sitting on your lunch break eating an overpriced ham and cheese croissant this is a real mood killer. For those of you who don't know (this included me at the time) The Royal Marsden hospital is the UK's leading Cancer treatment centre. My GP had rung me, following an appointment earlier in the day, to explain that all of her medical experience and training pointed to bone cancer and that was why I have been suffering with a pain in the top of my left leg since June 2018 (it's now December.) I don't remember much about the rest of the call apart from thinking I was now not hungry, which for me, was a rare experience. I sat staring at the wall thinking a thousand thoughts, most of which ended with my Mother. She died when I was eight – Spider Cancer, which originated from Breast Cancer. I have always been told that statistically I would get Cancer, but I did not expect that at twenty-nine. I threw the croissant in the bin (and of course properly recycled the paper bag it was in too.) I drifted through the rest of my café shift on cloud nine unable to focus. People gave their orders and I tapped at the till but my head was a million miles away. I kept thinking of what this meant going forward, how would I fight it and how sick I truly was? For the first time in a long time, I had nothing to say and was quiet and introverted. This sight would most likely be quite a pleasant image for most of my close friends.

I Finished work and walked home. The journey was about a mile. I always liked this walk as it was my own precious possession. I would fill it with podcasts, music or phone calls. Rain or shine I loved the solace of walking. Public transport in this country is far from calming. If you have ever been on a south west train you will understand my pain. Walking slower than normal (pain is kicking my ass) I ponder who to call and share the news with. The C bomb is one of the few words in the English dictionary that incites fear upon being breathed. It is one of the world's biggest killers earning its reputation with devastating consequences. Flicking through the familiar list of names on my phone in an out of body experience landed me on pressing the number for my father. The phone rang for a ridiculously long time and I prayed he would not pick up. "Hello Craig – How are you?" he answered, and I just went full blast into acting mode. Dad and I have set topics you see, which takes us over the elephant in the room that we haven't always got on. Rugby, football, work, his wife, lavish holidays and my sister. These safe subjects avoid feelings of emotion leaving us in safe territory. We were somewhere between the title race and how much I hated café life where I interrupted and told him I had received a phone call from my doctor. Telling a man who lost his wife to Cancer that their child may also suffer a similar fate was sobering. He did not say much apart from offering sporadic words of love. We agreed to tell no one, as nothing was concrete, and this was all speculation. I was due home in seven days for the annual Christmas celebration in the west country and knowing what this would do to my sister and stepmother was not worth considering. We set the rules of the pact and I went home to eat a meal I did not want to and to spend a night in bed staring at the ceiling, fulfilling every cliché of a T4 teen drama.

Two days later, I received a text message confirming my appointment referral at the Royal Marsden. That text burned the words into my mind. It was an automated message, so a computer had generated it. How interesting that a machine could publish words that could change someone's life forever. Following this, I went into full Google mode. If there was an article on the first two pages of my search (let's be honest no one goes further) then I was reading it. The good news was that bone Cancer was treatable, but this all depended on what stage we caught it at. It is amazing how quickly an event such as this brings the human mind into focus. I could see the blurred lines of life, but they were not of importance. I was going to fight this like my mother had. I was going to be a survivor and most importantly this would not define me.

Christmas arrived and the train journey home was quiet. My delightful employers had me in until 17:30pm on Christmas eve, so most people had done their travelling by now. Dad picked me up from the station and we went through our rehearsed pact again. I could see that this had shaken him to the core but did my best to lighten the mood. My sister had come earlier and was doing her normal routine of driving my step mum up the wall. Family politics never cease to amaze me. We all think our clan is the best and worst and we certainly don't think anyone has it as bad as me. The truth is, all families are mental. The arguing over the burnt toast or what TV channel to watch unites us in a performance of farcical behaviours. I arrived to find the house well-oiled and hungry as they had paused dinner for the prodigal son's return. We ate, we laughed, and all annoyed each other suitably. Classic Christmas eve shenanigans. Fast forward to about midnight and the last standing are my stepmother, old family friend and myself sipping something short and alcoholic and the bomb is dropped "Your father has been in an absurd mood – He is convinced you might have Cancer." There goes the pact.

The mixture of alcohol and emotions drove me into a monologue of confession. Neither of my audience said much after that. I think the term 'bum out' comes to mind in the curtain call of that evening. We agreed not to tell my sister as I wanted desperately to keep her happy over Christmas. Seeing her smile is still one of the most heart-warming things and listening to her chat rubbish infuriates me, such is the complications of sibling love. We got through to the 27th and I was back home and to work. The festive period had been a welcome distraction and despite the prolonged hangover, it was great to be with family. A few days later a letter arrived with an appointment to have an ultrasound scan. This was followed by a letter saying that the Royal Marsden did not except patients without said scans. This was understandable, as I imagine the wait to get into a centre of excellence is not short. I called the GP practice and asked why I had been refereed for an appointment without an Ultrasound? The receptionist went through the normal security questions of DOB and postcodes and gave no logical answer. It would seem my GP had dropped the ball. No one goes to the Royal

Marsden without an ultrasound, this a protocol and a logical one. Why would they see someone just on a hunch? I asked for an appointment with that specific GP to discuss this and I was told it was a three week wait. I left it and waited patiently for my Ultrasound like a duck looking at a rainy cloud.

I did not have Cancer. In fact, the scan showed nothing of any interest which could explain the worsening pain in my leg. I did not have a tumour or any issues with the bones and muscles in my leg, but the answers just threw up a hundred more questions. Why did I have this excruciating pain in the top of left leg and why was it getting worse? The quest for a resolution would be a radical one. My journey would take me through many appointments, dozens of healthcare professionals, countless scientific tests and living inside two hospitals. This book is my journey through the NHS and Private Healthcare systems and what happened along the way. I have changed the names, locations and details in respect to privacy but to those who figure out this simple code, I can only apologise.

A couple of weeks after my scan I found myself sat in front of the GP who had given a young man the sentence of Cancer a week before Christmas. Credit to her, she did apologise, she apologised profusely. I think she figured out that this set of events had not played out in a truly kosher way. It was not her fault in truth. There must be many people in this country whose lives are intact for the quick actions of GPs when they see something peculiar. I was lucky in the sense that Cancer was not my disease.

She told me I was being referred to the Spinal experts as now the leg was clear, a running thesis was emerging that could be to do with my back. This was good I thought, I was getting closer to meeting someone who could give me a definitive diagnosis. She would be putting the urgent label on it due to my severe pain. I politely asked how long it would take for my initial appointment to come through? "4-6 weeks" she replied. Wonderful I thought.

Limping Forward

Five weeks passed me by, and I was informed that I would have an appointment to see a physio at the hospital. I had presumed the referral was to see a spinal expert but an appointment was progress, so I held my tongue. My wait was made slower by resigning from the Café. By mid-January being on my feet for eight hours a day was impossible, and I was now unable to bend down without leaning on an aid. Simple tasks such as picking something off the floor now escaped me, leaving me moving like someone who had both hips replaced and was well over ninety. People who passed me in the street would sneak a glance which only makes you feel worse because I was losing all confidence in being mobile mainly down to my left leg having no strength in it.

Being male and under thirty, I did something without thinking of the consequences. Whilst I was fun-employed I continued to exercise. Running by now was off the table, only because my other half had served me a ban until a diagnosis was given. I decided to take up the watt bike in the garage. I had my days free, and so each morning I would do thirty minutes of cycling and pulling the alternate levers as hard as I could. For those of you who have not have this pleasure do try it but know that it knackers you out very quickly. I cannot express how stupid this was, but hindsight is a marvellous thing and these thirty minutes of exercise gave me an ounce of joy in a world of despair. I am being way too dramatic. The truth is I hate my body. Gone is the lean young man of yesterday and enter a twenty-nine-year-old with moobs and a swollen stomach. Cheeks rounded like a hamster holding his lunch all aided by Dominos and overpriced craft beer. For the last ten years I have been working on helping my inner voice love myself. No matter what I did, it would not change its discourse. Like a satanic Bart Simpson my conscious mumbled deprecating iterations and plagued my mind with self-doubt. This all lead me to doing exercise when I should have been resting my body. It hurt every time I got on and off the bike sponsored by my best mate at the time, co-codamol. The morning of the physio came, and I went on the bike first thing as I wanted them to see it's worse. Late afternoon my name was called and I limped off the plastic green chair into a room with a young lady in expensive neon Nike trainers and a white polo t-shirt on.

"I am not going to touch you" she mumbled. I have just spent the last forty minutes explaining my pain, it's history and how much it is affecting my life. I was expecting a slight physical examination at the very least. My heart sunk as we arrived at the next junction praying it was not a dead end. "You clearly have an issue with your spine. I am going to refer you to a spinal doctor." I am now very confused. My GP had suggested this was a spinal issue and that this appointment was with a back specialist. I did not know why I had just wasted my time going into detail with someone who was not going to prompt any affirmative action. I was angry and in pain. I wanted answers and wanted them all now. Despite my inner fury, I asked the physio politely why I was again being moved on with no diagnosis or treatment plan? The answer was to empty my heart of hope. She explained that this was to look at the spinal muscles but due to severity of the pain I was presenting with, she did not want to take some unnecessary chances. I think she got from my face that this was disheartening for me. I asked if there were any exercises or treatment I could pursue in the interim? She slowly explained that given the severity of my case, she would advise resting with gentle exercise. This was good news; the watt bike was helping after all. Maybe I was going to be a skinny model by summer and all my dreams would come true! She finished with saying the exercise should include walking and gentle swimming, but nothing strenuous. The referral would take 3-4 weeks and they would write to me in seven days to confirm this. I thanked her quietly and stumbled out of the hospital. I called my Dad and we skipped over the chit chat and I told him what had happened.

My father is a positive thinker. Problems are called challenges; books are for self-help and "winners never quit and quitters never win." A man in his seventies with an esteemed career behind him. His first job was cleaning toilets in a London hotel (he loves sharing this story) and he retired having owned two hotels and created the leading hospitality and leisure consultancy the UK has ever seen. A self-made man from Lincoln and my biggest fan. Life dealt him a couple of bad hands, but this never dampened his spirits. He supported two children as a single dad and we never went without. I am a huge admirer of him, although I don't tell him this enough. He sees life in black and white. He hates banks and how they screw the little people and uses his retirement threatening to take them all to local court for mischarges in his account which are usually under ten pounds. He is determined, aggressive and a born business entrepreneur who is was keen to see the sunlight in my perceived appointment of night.

"We know it is the back and that is a real win. We have ruled out the leg and muscular issues, which narrows down a long list of probable conditions." He was right, which pissed me off. I wanted to sulk and have a whinge, but he was determined to pitch rainbows all day. He reminded me that we also knew it was not Cancer and this turned my mind to thoughts of my mother. I would have been six when she was given her diagnosis, I cannot imagine what that must have been like for her or my Dad. His comment did lift me because whilst I had a limp and I was unable to run or bend down, I was alive and that was more than my late mum. I thanked my father and hung up. Riding on the bus back home and as I sat there a new thought emerged. I was not going to let this define me. I had been wasting away at home using my problems as an excuse to shut the world out. There are plenty of jobs that did not need me to mobile and I would find them. I got home, opened the laptop and started to search for local jobs in offices.

The recruitment buzz kept me entertained. Like a university fresher with Jager bombs I raced through applications with haste. Turns out there were plenty of office-based roles in my local area which were within hobbling distance to. In all the excitement of job hunting I had totally forgotten that a week had passed without any news on my appointment. The issue was I had no idea who to chase up as I had rushed out of the physio's company in a fluster. I went to my GP and asked the ever-helpful ladies on reception where I was heading next? They clicked and typed for a few moments and told me the people to call. I needed to contact the Integrated Care & Assessment Treatment Service (ICATS.) I rang the number and the phone was answered by a light Scottish accent. She could see my referral on the screen but informed me that no one had acted on it. If I had not called then nothing would have progressed. This really pissed me off. It felt like I was the only one who cared about getting this resolved. I again wanted to lash out but held my tongue and remembered it was not the Scottish lady's fault, even if I wanted to recreate a scene from Macbeth with her. Good manners prevailed and she confirmed another appointment with the doctor at my local hospital which was to investigate my spinal issues. This was a big win as it was only six days away. A few short days before a possible diagnosis. To make things even better, I also landed a job that week. My father's good vibes were flooding in and for the first time in a while, I felt motivated. My new job was challenging but in a good way and I was a little closer of solving the Agatha Christie novel unravelling in my spine.

"We are going to need an MRI scan to tell us more" the Spinal doctor told me. The Magnetic Resonance Imaging Machine would show my spine in all its glory and offer the final verdict on my pain. However, keys to the kingdom would come at a cost, payment of a four week wait. It is now February and I have been on this path a long time, another pause seemed agonising. I asked the doctor for advice with pain management, he suggested seeing my GP. This made me smile, as I had images of walking out of that meeting with any number of tropical diseases but wrote it down anyway to look attentive. He said I should be on medication for nerve pain as he thinks that is the source of the problem. He did not offer any more on this but I could see the light at the end of the tunnel. The idea of a back problem was not new to me. When I was sixteen I fractured a vertebrate in my spine playing rugby for my beloved Avon RFC. It was in a cup final and my injury paused the game which my team mates went on to lose. I had spent time in a back brace and had injections in my spine afterwards. I asked if this was linked to my current situation and I was relived it was not as the pain was in the wrong part of my spine. A small relief to know that whatever was hindering me was a new foe and one that would take more than a tubi-grip and a couple of paracetamols. I left the hospital feeling a little more in the know and thanked the doctor. He would see me after the scan and would in fact be the person to diagnose my issue.

I called the MRI desk the following morning to be greeted by a panicked voice. The MRI machine at my local hospital had been down for three days due to a fault. This meant that all appointments were being pushed back. My scan had been labelled with an urgent request but even with this it equalled a 6 week wait. Here is where I faced the first NHS vs Private standoff.
The waiting times available to me were the following:

6 Weeks via NHS
or
2 days and £299 via Private Healthcare.

Three hundred quid for a photograph of your spine is ridiculous. Comparatively, a picture of Kim Kardashian's spine for that price would be bargain. As you may have guessed I did not possess private healthcare insurance, so it was hard cash from my own pocket. This is the brilliant business model of private healthcare. On a normal day when you are pain free and have no worrying symptoms, paying hundreds of pounds for a scan is laughable, but I was in the other corner. I have been living with this getting worse for eight months and it has been three and a half months since I asked for a Doctor's opinion. I was tired, angry, frustrated and fed up. I had done my waiting through Cancer scares, physio and spinal specialists and this scan was the very thing that would answer all the big questions, this was the last step. Therefore you pay if it is a pound or a million quid, if you have the means you don't have a choice. My life was being turned upside down. My manager has asked me twice why I keep taking tablets so frequently and always sighed in pain when I get up from my chair. I couldn't run. I couldn't bend down. I could barely walk without someone thinking I was Kaiser Sozay. I phoned up, gave them my doctor's name with my credit card details and I had an appointment two days later.

You always know when you're in a private clinic because there is a free coffee machine. They never tend to make the best coffee; however, I strongly endorse their mochas.

A sweet blend of drinking chocolate and watered-down espresso is such treat, especially when waiting on a healthcare appointment. Giving you free caffeinated drinks surely makes it value for money, doesn't it? One week later I am back with the spinal doctor who smiles at me when he calls my name in the waiting area. This is going to be good news; a smile is secret code for a clear scan I thought as I limped slowly into his office. He sat me down and was kind and compassionate whilst he gave me the words, I had craved to hear for eight months:

"You have two bulging discs. This is where the discs in your spine are poking out or prolapsed. They are compressing the nerves that run down the back of your left leg which is why you are in so much pain. The two vertebrates are L4 & L5. There are three options that are available to you now: The first is Physio but given the length of time you have suffered I think this would be ineffective. Second is a steroid injection into the base of your spine which may help with the pain but does not reduce the bulges. Last but not least is surgery. We would cut into your spine and remove pieces of the vertebrate, freeing the compressed nerves and hopefully all the pain that goes with it." Think of the disc as a jam doughnut (custard flavour if you're a ledge) and think of that being squeezed. This pressure causes your filling of choice to ooze out. Where the thick and creamy filling spills out it touches the nerve and forces it against its will (like bending a twig without breaking it.) This angers the long twig that runs down my left leg and causes a pain that feels like a sharp razor slashing with a warm throbbing sensation which is aggressively cooking you alive or a pain that occupies your mind so much you become a grumpy and short-tempered prat.

I was overwhelmed but I can remember I started to smile uncontrollably, which the doctor must have thought quite peculiar. Sherlock has left the building ladies and gentlemen. Case closed and we can all go home. I declared that I wanted to have surgery as in my hyperactive mind it seemed the only logical choice. Cut the thing out and away we go. I'll be back running in no time. Spine guy said the magic words "you can expect a 3-4 week wait for an appointment" and this time he was speaking the truth. I did not care at all with this information. All the fear of the unknown was removed. I had been diagnosed and it was treatable. For the following days, it was like I forgot the pain I was in. I went to work with a sense of calm knowing that a quick operation and all would be fine. Phycology is fascinating, as my pain seemed easier after the big reveal. A little bit of my confidence had come back. A week later I headed to work in London to attend a conference in Canary Wharf. On my way home as I entered the underground station I collapsed as my left leg had given way in being able to support my body weight. I fell over and lay on the concrete floor in agony waiting for somebody to notice as I tried to figure out why I could not feel my left leg anymore. My honeymoon period was well and truly over.

Enter Hospital

Staring at the ceiling of Canary Wharf underground station I could certainly empathise with Natalie Imbruglia. I was torn between getting up or just staying still in hope of the ground swallowing me up. Neither of these came to play as a wonderful woman who works for TFL rushed over to assist me. A small circle had formed around me and I remember catching the eyes of a man in a delightful navy suit who slowed his walking pace but did not stop. Miss TFL asked me a few basic questions and I muttered some answers back. I reached into my blazer pocket and swallowed double the normal dose of co-codamol (I do not condone this action, but you have to believe me, it was an emergency.) She helped me to my feet, and I checked to see if I could now put weight on my left leg. I walked a few steps in a *Walking Dead* audition style and figured although the pain was immense, I could feel my leg, even if it had strange sensations rushing up and down. I felt like a sparkler was being held down and dragged along my nerve which felt very bizarre. I thanked the lady and refused her offer to call an ambulance. The very last thing I wanted was to be stranded in a central London Hospital, as it was far from home and unfamiliar. My phone was not cracked so that was a highlight but as I descended underground my mind began to race with what on earth was happening in my left leg.

The journey home had enough length and trepidation to become a trilogy of films. I hobbled through stations and trains, never being offered a seat, collecting stares of strangers pondering why I was moving in such a peculiar fashion? I arrived at my local station and got a lift to hospital by my partner's mother. Unsurprisingly, the accident and emergency department was busy, and the neon screen indicated a waiting time of two hours. Crossing the threshold into a hospital always fills me with emotions. I take a quick glance around the waiting room and assess how bad my problems are compared to the others? A woman holds a bandage to a bloodied hand, a younger woman is complaining of sickness which she thinks derives from a skiing tumble and a young boy will not stop crying much to the delight of his parents. Waiting rooms are tiny microcosms of society. Health has never discriminated, and this setting confirms it. Walking up to the desk I am greeted by someone with a sharp tone of voice:

Sharpie: How can I help you?
Me: My leg, it is gone.
Sharpie: What do you mean gone? Do you have any sensation in it?
Me: Yes, but it is abnormal.
Sharpie: Can you feel it?
Me: Yes but/
Sharpie: / You can walk on it?
Me: Barely
Sharpie: What help would you like?
Me: I have two bulged discs in my vertebrate.
Sharpie: How do you know that?
Me: A doctor told me last week.
Sharpie: Where?
Me: Here.
Sharpie. Right. Can you pass Urine?

Me: I don't know. I have not tried, I collapsed at/
Sharpie: /Are you having any treatment for your back?
Me: Yes, I have an appointment with/
Sharpie: / I will put you to see one of the doctors.
Me: Thank you.
Sharpie: Please take a seat.

This conversation passed by in a flash and I felt I had just been interrogated rather than checked in. No blame to Sharpie as I am sure I was one of many customers who all present cryptic symptoms and to be fair she looked very tired and stressed. I made it to the nearest chair and slumped down, switching positions like a toddler every ten seconds to create comfort. The pills I had swallowed must have kicked in as the pain was duller in my leg but still had the sparkler party going on. I tried to read a magazine and then count the people in the room. I have often created strange mind games to distract myself. Counting, talking to myself or imagining passing cars can fly up and down on command by my blinking. Everyone in here has a baffling facial expression of pain, stress or discomfort. I ponder how many of these people are actually fitting of an emergency department? Then this condemning narrative is placed upon my shoulders and I imagine I am wasting everyone's time. The NHS is stretched as it is, I know what is wrong and I probably need a few days off my feet to help the bugles relax a little. The self-accusations are interrupted by my name being called. An hour and a half, the screen had lied. I take one last glance around the room and followed Doctor Parker into a room.

This man was worth the wait. He listened keenly as I described my history and recent calamity. He seemed interested, concerned and compassionate all at the same time. This relaxed me into a sense of calm. By this time my partner had arrived also and sat with me silent but supportive. Next up was the physical examination. These were never my favourite experiences and varied much from the same scenario depicted in hundreds of Adult films. 'The stroke' (checking sensation on each shin by running fingers along it) confirmed that the nerve in my left leg was not responsive and clocked a 40% sensation in comparison to the right which was 100%. 'The mega stroke' (similar to the stroke except the sensation is around one's back passage) revealed a full 100% in feeling which was good in relation to a working spine. Last came 'the squeeze' (still in the rear end, but I will let your imagination reveal what this may entail) and that also was felt 100%. Lastly, he asked if I could pass Urine and still had sensation around my groin (luckily this was only a vocal inspection.) The reason for this line of inquiry was that if any of these tests were 0% or no it meant that something was unstable in my spine, or the bulging discs had exploded or any number of extreme possibilities that would have required very urgent attention. The tests had revealed two things. The pressure on my leg was getting worse. The vertebrates were still stable, and I would not require emergency surgery. I took this as good news.

Parker then enquired what my next steps were? I told him I had an appointment with Mr Quiet (spoiler alert) in ten days and he was a spinal surgeon who fingers crossed, was going to sort me good and proper. He then stated that his course of action was a simple one: get me through to that appointment without any more major incidents. He prescribed a few more drugs including an old friend of mine called the suppository. He did so in such delicate language that when he left the room to get one for me my girlfriend had no idea: "Really? He is going to put a pill up your ass?" After a quick debrief and now understanding fully what was to happen, she had the love to pull the blue curtain around my bed and sit just out of sight. The doctor returned with a chaperone (safeguarding at its finest) which included a young lady standing over me and watched him lube me up and do the deed, twice. I cracked a tasteless joke as he handed me some Tramadol followed by a slip for more supplies. We shook hands (yes, he has washed them by now) and I went on my way. Life had caught up with me finally and I was to slow everything right down. No watt bike, work (until after the weekend) and long travels to Canary Wharf. It was now the end of March, and my bulges had gone from a twinge to stopping me from walking (if only for a short period.) Despite my efforts to ignore that I had a serious health issue, the body had finally won. I text my boss and explained the evening's events. I told her that I would not be work tomorrow but would be back in action on Monday. My wonderful girlfriend drove me home as I started to feel normal again. The skittles in my behind were performing miracles and I collapsed into bed, exhausted by the day's events.

By Sunday, things were not getting any better. My leg was going from bad to worse. The sparklers seemed to be flashing on and off in my leg paired with sharp pains and instability when I stood up or walked. On the advice of my girlfriend we went back to the hospital as Parker had duly noted, "if it gets worse you know where we are." I wonder if this more of a "have a nice day" sentence than an actual invitation. They have to say it as it rounds the treatment off but I honestly think they would prefer we didn't come back, especially as in theory there was nothing practical they could do. Despite this growing paranoia I went back to the waiting room of delights. Much to my disappointment, Sharpie was not on the desk and it was a man in red robes. Crimson quizzed me and asked the usual questions about sensations, urine passing and pain. He said I would be rushed through and within thirty minutes I was back in front of a doctor. Doctor Quiet Junior was an orthopaedic specialist who had trained under Mr Quiet who I was due to see shortly. He explained that based on how I walked towards him he was not going to admit me. Quiet Junior also added that he would up the drugs. We were heading to the Premier League by method of Morphine. I had once been acquainted with this powerful aliment and although it relieves pain it also sends you floating through the stratosphere. He advised me that work was not a good idea and to keep things as minimal as possible which I hated. Work was the distraction keeping me from losing my mind. I did not want to be stuck at home, on strong drugs worrying about my back, or leg or whatever else was going wrong with me. My new job had been positive for me and was a career opportunity going places. I wanted to keep on trying to make an effort in life and not just give up because it was a little difficult. It was just pain but when it occupies your mind it transforms the way you think and feel. Your patience is taken, mind plagued with doubts and most of all I turned into a horrible person to be around. Pissed off and muttering under my breath I shook Quiet Junior's hand and took the slip for my super drugs. My girlfriend was optimistic and did her best to cheer me up, but I was slowly turning within myself and ignoring everything happening on the exterior.

The morphine did not help in the slightest. I was expecting it to at least touch the sides of the pain. It did, however, make me drowsy, constipated and relaxed to the point of being seven pints deep (that's right, I can drink seven all by myself.) I was also taking nerve drugs before I went to sleep. They are very peculiar and make you sleep as if you are in a coma only to wake up the next day with a feeling in your head as if the ground you walk on is made entirely of clouds. I would not recommend these to anyone who needed to be awake for work which was certainly not me. Mixed in with the drugs was the deepening realisation that my life was falling apart. Moving around was difficult and painful and being on all the drugs made me feel as if I was not really there. On Wednesday, I visited my therapist loaded on the new cocktail. She immediately remarked "what has happened to you?" as she instantly observed something was very different in my energy.

I have been seeing a therapist since September last year. Following me leaving a graduate scheme I was badly suited for I had a mini mental breakdown. I was medicated for depression and anxiety and for the first time in my life I lost total confidence in myself. The real reason I did not seek a doctor for so long about my leg was that I was intent on keeping my progress on an upward trend and not accept that I could be on my way out again. I had gone from unemployment to café to junior HR role and now back to unemployment. I had tried and failed. Whilst I was making my way through all the noise I have written so far; I was in constant dialogue with my therapist. Granted I did not attend every week (which she loved to mention) but when I arrived it was for the better. We covered a range of topics including my Mother's passing, my family, the graduate scheme, life in general and looking back, my leg. We spoke a lot about my leg, but I always seemed convinced it was no big deal and a resolution beckoned. Talking about your feelings and experiences truly can work wonders and would honestly recommend everyone seeks therapy. Unfortunately for me, this therapist could not heal my worsening leg, that would take a different set of skills entirely.

My normal optimism was gone on that Wednesday and it was written all over my face. That, or she noticed I was off my face on opiate pain killers. After her question rung out around the room, I explained the events of the last seven days which had included the Canary collapse, rounded off with two separate visits to hospital. She thanked me for coming realising this would have been a monumental struggle. I had been driven to the door, so that made life a little clearer. She then commented that work when I am chemically induced is not the best practice, but we chatted about how crap I felt. I don't remember what I talked about for the rest of the session except for the ending. Figuring the leg of doom would worsen I requested a pause in our work. She happily agreed and regrettably that was the last time I saw my therapist in person.

A week on from the Canary Collapse and the pain was unbearable. I woke up and made my way downstairs where my girlfriend's mum was making a coffee. We spoke about how bad things were and she mentioned returning to my favourite hospital which I politely declined and left to have a shower. After washing I sat on the bed to put my jeans on and I couldn't. I tried slowly but my leg was having none of it. The pain was off the chart, the leg was not able to straighten or bend properly and with that I gave up. The leg had won, and I was not going to fight the pain anymore. Barely able to walk, I made it downstairs and asked for help dressing and that I needed to get back to hospital as quickly as possible.

As Elphaba famously sung: "Something has changed within me, something is not the same." This is all that kept flooding my mind, meaning my leg issues not *Wicked* the musical, as I entered the hospital through the usual entrance. No crimson or Sharpie but a nice young lady who we can call Glinda for now. I knew the drill by now and stated that my leg was worsening, I had sensations in my groin, I could pass urine and what medication I was on. Glinda looked surprised at my monologue but smiled warmly. "Been here before?" she asked, "Third time in a week" I replied. To my fairy Godmother's credit, she quickly tapped away at her magical keyboard and I was in front of a new doctor inside ten minutes.

Doctor Topman asked what had changed and I replied "everything." What I meant by that seems very over the top, which is classic me. Up until that morning I was willing to fight the pain and keep it in a box whilst going about my daily tasks. I was happy with the limp, inability to bend or stretch and general discomfort in my life. The human body is an incredible coping mechanism. The fact we are still here proves that but mine was failing. Not being able to dress myself brought it all home nine months after my leg first fizzled a little. Off stump is flying out of the ground and the worst thing is I knew exactly where the ball would pitch. The detail and dismay I expressed was certainly over Topman's pay grade, but he listened keenly. I finished my sermon and then he said they were going to get me seen by the orthopaedic doctors. They showed me to another waiting room passed the magnetic doors and sat me down.

If I was about to enter hell, this was the waiting room for it. In everyone's favourite game of which patient is worst off, I was losing this round. A young woman in a grey hoodie looked in agony opposite a woman in a wheelchair who was trembling and pale. As I was taking in my surroundings something started to happen in my spine which did not feel good at all. My back started to spasm paired with shooting pains of a javelin being thrust the inside of the leg. I was moving sporadically in my chair and everything in the room went blurry. In hindsight, I realise now I had taken no pain medication that morning, it would seem the morphine was working, because it was stopping me feeling this. My girlfriend's mother was still sat with me and now was up at the desk as I entered a sort

33

of fit. Doctor Mean arrived and ushered me into a room. I was bobbing up and down as if the seat were hot. I was in agony. I screamed out in desperation as he poked and examined. I begged him to stop but understood the essential nature of the inspection. He told me that I would be admitted for 'pain management.' I had no idea what that meant but I remember being relieved as the pain was taking me out of my mind. Lastly, he tried to get me to walk and like the Canary Collapse I could not put any weight on my left leg and attempting it caused an indescribable shooting pain. I fell back onto the bed and lay flat. Doctor Mean muttered something I did not hear and left. That confirmed it, I was moving into hospital for the indefinite future.

I asked my girlfriend's mother to leave me to it as it would not be long before I was seen to. I had my book and a white wall to stare at to keep me amused. She checked one more time and took her exit. Then it was quiet. Laying on the bed flat was the only position where the pain was controllable. I was gagging for my pain medication and when the nurse came in with a paracetamol it broke my heart. Requesting my regular medication was now not possible without a doctor's signature and there were none around. The best they could do was a co-codamol instead of the paracetamol. Realising this was my best option I thanked the nurse and then asked her what the next steps were. "You are being admitted here. We need to wait until a bed is available on the correct ward and once this is done, we will take you up. It should not be long and please let me know if you need anything." Waiting all alone and the world seemed to slow the spin. Thoughts of what was to come raced across my mind like flaming comets paired with self-critique of why I had let things get so out of control. Yet again my life was falling to pieces and in truth I was sick of it. Being honest, as the whitewashed walls of the NHS hospital strangled my consciousness like a tightening brace I prayed the noise would stop and peace could engulf me. Don't really know how to unpack that but at the time it was crystal clear.

Beds are very popular, and hence I had a long waiting time. I spent 6 hours staring at the wall before being wheeled up to my ward, the home of orthopaedic and post operation patients. I sat on my bed in a room of five other beds and looked around nervously. A few had tubes attached to them, the smell of something foreign lingered in the air and I was drowning in an overwhelming feeling of vulnerability. A couple of nurses settled me into bed with a cup of tea and an open heart. Throughout all of my stay I have been overwhelmed by the hard work and compassion of the nursing team, which in this dark room on a foreign mattress was worth its weight in gold. I rolled around and tried to settle for a sound night's sleep, how fruitless this effort would be. Some moments later, the man next to me started to shout something in a tone that cut through your ears and stabbed you in the brain: "He is smoking, that man, over there! I've just had an operation and that selfish prick is smoking inside the ward!!!

Settling In

Startled by the man's screaming I was suddenly overwhelmed by the smell of rich cigarette smoke. I assumed this had crept into our air space through an open window or air vent. "You're fucking smoking!" screamed my neighbour, and he continued to scream profanities until the nurses on night duty ran in. Whilst this was going on, the patient in the corner of the room was making a heck of a racket clambering around and quickly jumping back into bed. The nurses burst into our room:

Night Nurse: What's going on?

Screaming man: He's fucking smoking!

Night Nurse: Who is?

Screaming man: That man in the corner. He has been smoking in our room. I am trying to recover from a stomach operation and that selfish prick is smoking. He is risking all our health. Get him taken out of here now!

Night Nurse: Calm down my love, I am sure he is not….

Night Nurse is now in the corner of the room by the open window. She can see ash all over the ledge and can now smell what we smell and that's the stench of smoke which has been circulating around the room. Smokey (the patient by the window) is lying very still. To explain the room, there are three beds on each side of our small abode. The beds are divided by flimsy blue paper curtains and there is one window in the back-left corner where Smokey has set up camp. Screaming man and I occupy the right side with total view of the window and the next set of actions. Upon Night Nurse discovering the evidence she made the quick deduction that Smokey was the culprit. She begins her line of enquiry:

Night Nurse: Did you just smoke a cigarette inside this room?

Smokey: No.

Night Nurse: If you are not responsible, how did this ash get here? Where is that smell of smoke coming from?

Smokey: I have no idea. I was just sitting here having a sleep, I've no idea what this is all about!!

Screaming man: He is a liar. He was just up smoking outside the window. Get him out of this ward. NOW!

Smokey: I am not going to admit to something I didn't do. I have no idea how that ash got there, and smoke must be from outside.

Night Nurse was in a difficult position. The culprit was a blind faced liar and she had a room full of sick people having witnessed this idiot smoking. She opened his cupboard to find a lighter and pack of cigarettes to which Smokey continued to deny his crime. She confiscated the contraband and gave him a stern telling off. Smokey followed his reprimand with empty promises of good behaviour and Night Nurse left the room. Screaming man then kicked off and started a barrage of foul language and threats of legal action. He wanted Smokey removed as he saw him as risk for his rest and recuperation. He could do little more than scream as his recent operation had left him unable to get up. He accused Night Nurse of accepting foul play, being soft and was very aggressive in his vocabulary. Night Nurse absorbed every word and left again. Screaming man eventually ran out of air and went silent, but his panting was evidence of his exhaustion.

Smokey lay quietly knowing he was caught red handed and had just made enemies of five very sick men. I sat there silent through the whole event in true fascination and disgust. The selfish actions of Smokey were inexcusable, but I can see Night Nurse had little power. You cannot kick a sick man from his hospital bed in the middle of the night and discharging patients is a long game of cat and mouse which takes hours. I felt sorry for that woman who took the abuse from Screaming Man and the disrespectful and hollow lies from Smokey. She didn't deserve any of this, especially as she had and would continue to care for these patients.

Oxygen is a very common aide to many patients in hospital and is an extremely flammable gas. Apart from the fact it is illegal to smoke inside a hospital, had one of Smokey's sparks met some of the O2 the entire room would have gone up in a fantastic fireball. I cannot imagine that Smokey had considered this aspect of his midnight blow out but I was relieved that none of this had come to play. Despite my silence, I was furious that this had happened. In my silent state of shock, I looked up on my phone how to lodge an official complaint to the hospital. The internet came up trumps and had an official form. I logged the whole incident in detail and left nothing out. I clicked submit and then was welcomed by a page that summed up the strain on our beloved NHS: *Thank you for your submission. We aim to reply to all complaints within 35 working days.* I put my phone on the side and attempted to fall asleep in my hazy hospital room.

The next morning, I was woken at about 6:00am which was to become my routine for the next few weeks. First up are the healthcare assistants who come around to do your observations before handover. These included, checking your temperature, blood pressure and sugar levels. The primary focus of these regular checks is for infection which can lead to Sepsis. If any of these checks are irregular it is a quick indicator that something is not right in your body. Temperature probes are stuck in your ear; blood pressure squeezes your upper arm in an inflatable strap and glucose levels are stuck on the end of your index finger. These tests are minimally invasive and after a couple of days you get very used to them. All of the results are written neatly on your chart as they whizz onto the next patient.

After observation come morning drugs. These are the last ones done by the night nurses before they leave to be replaced by the day team. Most Nurses work in shifts of twelve hours and this is usually eight to eight. Post drug hand out is handover. This is where the night team go around each bed with the day team and explain any changes from normal but also a brief summary of why that patient is in hospital. These feel a little intimidating. On that first morning, I was running on very little sleep and in a foul mood. Enter a huddle of twelve people who go into detail about my condition and what is being done. I listened intently and then corrected one of them as they claimed I was here for back pain "The pain is in my leg, but it is caused by a problem in my spine." As the sentence left my mouth, I regretted my words immediately. Everyone looked at me and a nurse in a dark blue uniform just reassured me that everything was ok that they were going to take good care of me. I cannot express how valuable kindness is in this environment. Having been brought in the night before I had little time for introductions and a quick tour. I had no idea who was in charge, where I was (apart from the label on the wall) or what course of treatment they were going to pursue. The lady in the navy turned out to be a sister on the ward. A sister is a senior nurse and in a position of authority on the ward. The sister who had calmed me with a few words was sister Navy. After I was finished grabbing the spotlight in handover, the welcome committee left me to once again be all alone. Waking up in hospital is a strange sensation of unfamiliar surroundings and pain, for me it will always be about pain. My mind was plagued with what this pain was and how much damage it was doing to my body. Being in that bed in a room full of people you truly feel all alone.

Last in the morning routine, and the most important, is Oli. This young man would wheel a steel trolley bed to bed offering tea, coffee or 'choccy woccy do dah'

(Smokey's nickname for the hot chocolate sachets.) My order was a black coffee with an extra spoon of coffee in it. I needed this to get me over the nerve drug hangover and I always felt as if it kept me aware and on my toes. Smokey's order was a 'choccy woccy do dah' which translates to a hot chocolate with three extra spoons of sugar. Before living in hospital, I had never met anyone who added sugar to drinking chocolate and would often ponder if it gave him superpowers, the immense ability to be Smokey in all his glory. Smokey would follow his morning beverage with a walk downstairs and outside to have a smoke and pick up his daily reading material *The Sun* newspaper. He has a broken ankle and a broken wrist. He cannot use crutches or a wheelchair but has a Zimmer frame with wheels on. He is incredibly mobile for someone with such injuries but for all I knew maybe it wasn't just chocolate he was drinking. Oli was always smiling, talkative and a mate. He was a Bournemouth supporter and attended most home games as his father wrote a popular blog about the club. By the third morning he would automatically bring me my drink and on the occasional event when I was so out of it I missed this entire early routine, I would wake to find my hot drink on my tray in front of me. Getting to know Oli was a real highlight as no matter how crap I felt, his conversations would take me to a place of serene calm, if only for a few moments. It is also worth noting that Oli was a big Star Wars fan and this is a real bonus given that the Skywalker Saga is life.

If you were lucky and on my first morning I was, after breakfast you would receive a visit from one of the doctors. Upon Doctor Mean's arrival, I was glad to see a familiar face. Without any explanation or introduction, he launched into a direct passage that explained I would be visited by the pain team who would work on managing my discomfort. Alongside this I had my appointment with Mr Quiet in five days in this very hospital and we would be continuing Doctor Parker's mission of getting me there without incident (kind of.) In my naive state, I asked about my mobility having not quite realised the seriousness of my situation. Dr Mean told me the Physio team would also be along to coach me on that side of things. He then left in a puff of smoke leaving more questions than answers.

Oli returned and asked me what I would like to eat for breakfast. He replied they had prunes, cereal, toast and beans. I hoped this was not a smoothie. I was not hungry by any case but to avoid hassle from every nurse in your ward one must eat, even if it feels like stuffing an overflowing bin with one more beer bottle. Food choices are done the day before. Three cute menus for each square meal of the day. You had the choice to tick one item from each section and were reminded of this in bold. Smokey had discovered a different tactic, he would tick as many boxes as possible and sit in hope that the catering Gods would hear his cry for help. Some days his tray would arrive brimming with food. For a man, quite slight he could certainly handle his nosh.

I took a slow breath and looked around my room. Smokey was enjoying some toast in a loud crunching motion spreading crumbs airborne. Screaming man was quiet this morning but we don't judge as the poor bloke had endured a rough night. Gerry, opposite me was still asleep snoring like a fog horn and then my thought went back in myself like a reverse cough. This was to be home for now and it was nothing like the glamourous Holby City. It was scary, cold and overwhelming. I drew a sharp breath and my eyes welled up because I was a long way from Kansas and could see no hope of a way back home.

Through the Curtains

The one thing about sharing a room with five other men is that all that separates us is thin blue paper curtains. They are retractable and pulled close when anyone needs a 'private' conversation. We hear everything about each other's lives from doctor's updates to heart felt conversations between loved ones. The wash of blue is drawn, and all is out in the open but we all ignore this when the curtains reopen as if we heard nothing. We behave as the stereotypical British person: nosy as hell, but very polite about it.

After the antics of the first evening Smokey was not winning any popularity awards. He was ignored by all of us after the cigarette incident and you could see this bothered him. Comradery in the ward is strong and although we all have our issues; chit chat is part of the daily routine. These can range from news headlines to whole life stories. The one thing no one spoke about was the reality of their illness or condition. I was the youngest in the room on my second day which would often pull amusing comments from my seniors with remarks 'you're too young to be in here.' I wish that that were true but given my current mobility I was moving more like a pensioner than a man in the dying embers of his twenties. Talking to Gerry, opposite me was a warming exchange. We were both being treated by the physios to help us move better and would often joke about who would win in a foot race of us both using frames. Gerry was deep into his eighties but had lived a busy life. He has been based in Africa for his work and spoke proudly of his travels. He had a daily visit from his wife who was the most glamorous woman I have ever seen. She would rock up with immaculate hair, colour coded outfits and loud jewellery. After a few visits, she would come and spend a few moments on my side of the room just asking polite questions about my interests and career. I hugely treasured Gerry and his wife as they had lived a long life with fifty years of marriage but still conversed as lovesick teenagers. I would also often be on the receiving end of Gerry's wife baking skills as one of the ward rituals was the delivery of her baked delights. I never had the stomach to eat them, but always forced a few nibbles in to be polite. Gerry and his visitors never drew the blue curtain as if their conversation was welcome for all to join and I often did which provided a happy distraction from the realities of the ward.

About mid-morning on my third day a smartly dressed woman who I later learn is a social worker comes to talk to Smokey. Curtains drawn, and the through early exchanges I learn that Smokey has recently been in prison for drunk driving and is on probation. He has a wife and two children, neither of whom he sees anymore. He is a self-proclaimed alcoholic and has aroused suspicion that he may be drinking inside the hospital. Smokey is homeless and although he has family, they all refuse to house him. The social worker explains that Smokey is near to being discharged and that the local council are looking to find him emergency housing. Smokey protests his injury (a broken ankle and wrist caused from a drunken fall) are hospital worthy and he has a right to be here. He is made to blow into a breathalyser which draws

0.0%. He then explodes into a long monologue of how his life has fallen apart, booze had saved him and following that, destroyed him. Trying to rebuild his life he desperately wants a safe place to live (away from addicts) and a chance to get his families trust back. The social worker is quiet and absorbs his testimony. She is polite in her reassurance to get Smokey back on track and takes her cue to leave.

This exchange made me think. Had I judged Smokey too soon for his smoking inside? When I saw him bundling about clutching a *Sun newspaper* and half his teeth missing maybe I did think the worst but the first night's antics did nothing to support his character. As I am deep in my mind the tea trolley is pushed in. Oli, who would have an optimistic outlook on life even after a world-wide nuclear holocaust, approaches Smokey and simply asks "can I get you anything to drink?" With this question Smokey teared up and gently replied with a request for his usual hot chocolate with three sugars in it. This gesture of kindness touched him, and Smokey started to rant about his problems with no filter. As if Oli had now become the social worker the young man listened keenly, smiled and then offered him some biscuits. Smokey chose the custard creams and thanked him for listening. How cathartic a hot drink can be. We all thought differently about Smokey after that. The context of his life had been exposed but gave reasoning for his behaviour (almost.) We started to accept him again in our playful ward jokes and discussion of football players and wanker politicians. I had learned not to judge so quickly and understand that in this place we were all equal, on the same bed, with a childlike vulnerability holding out a trembling hand in desperate need for care.

Fast forward to about eleven that evening, and I make my way on crutches to the bathroom which had previously been occupied by Smokey. The room stank and I quickly discovered the source of the odour. Peeking from the bin were three crushed empty cans of Foster's lager. I sighed and then emptied my bladder. Limping back to my bed I spotted Smokey receiving his tablets of morphine, the dessert to his entree of beer and thought how sad this man must be inside to act in such a destructive way. Not everyone in a hospital wants to get better or even to leave and for Smokey, life seemed very good right now.

Knowing everything about your neighbours can be a welcome distraction to your day. I have met a variety of men with different injuries and issues. One man I spent eight days living with me had a monumental effect on me to which I will never forget, his name was Todd. He arrived on the ward cursing the nurses and hospital porters around him whilst flamboyantly waving his arms around in the air. He was clearly in huge pain and shrieked insults and demands. When they parked him up he looked around at us and had that look of disappointment, like the one you give the waiter when they bring you the wrong thing on the menu and you want to scream and break things but you just scowl instead. Todd looked around and then looked down and passed out in exhaustion from his energetic entrance. Todd is in his sixties and has tubes in both arms and bag for his urine and a bag for his poo. He is wrinkled, with a few odd hairs on his head. I imagined he was successful in life and I judged this entirely by his designer wash bag. Green leather and a gold zip. Pure class. I imagine Todd buys suits from Saville Row and reads the *Financial Times*. Todd also has an American wife named Janice who is a tour de force. Raised on the east coast with red and black hair, she is intimidating and oozing with confidence – A woman to keep Todd in line.

Day two of living with Todd and he called me over to his bed. "What on earth are you up to wearing those, bit loud aren't they?" He was commenting on my tartan pyjamas (Ralph Lauren, naturally) which I had always cherished. We laughed and enjoyed this humour. We then chatted about a few things and upon reaching the topic of cricket shared stories of being at Lords for a test match. During our chat, Janice arrived and joined in. I told her I lived in New York once upon a time and she told me of all the flats she had occupied in Manhattan. She carried great pride in stating she was an 'East Coast Girl' which I loved. A few trump gags were made, and my time was up as the daily nurse rounds had begun.

Just as lights off began that evening, Todd started being sick all over himself. When the lights went on, we could see it was a deep crimson colour (like a rich red wine) but this was because it had blood in it. Looking at it seemed intrusive, but Todd's vomiting was so loud and aggressive it woke everyone up. Gerry pressed the emergency buzzer by his bed and screamed for some help. This felt bad and the doctors soon came up and took him away for various tests.

When Todd came back it was pretty grim. The doctors drew those bloody blue curtains and told him he had a cancerous tumour in his stomach which was inoperable. The rouge in his sick was caused by bleeding in the stomach. In real talk: he had a few weeks to live. The air hung like a heavy cloud. The room was silent and the gravity of what had been said smashed everyone over the head with a cricket bat. The doctors then said a few sentences that nobody heard, opened the curtains and left. What followed the next few days was Janice going to war with everyone she spoke with to get her husband home as quickly as possible. This took many phone calls, blunt requests and quiet threats but after a day or so all parties were happy, Todd was going home to be comfortable in familiar surroundings. The way Janice had managed the situation was with precision and gumption. I cannot fathom how hard it was for her to be making arrangements for her husband to go home because he is on borrowed time. Her actions could only be defined with selfless love and living to the scared promise 'in sickness and in health, until death do us part."

On the morning of his discharge I was leaving to have my pre-surgery assessment. I wanted to go over and speak to Todd and Janice before I went. I limped over with my crutches and spoke. I can't really remember what I said but what followed I'll never forget:

Todd: Do you know who Noel coward is?"

Me: Yes of course.

Todd: He has a saying which I want you to remember 'be whatever you like, just don't be boring.'

I was done. The tears came from my eyes sprinting down my cheek. I touched his arm and muttered a "thank you." I turned to Janice and hugged her knowing these next few weeks would be the worst of her days and parted company with a soft goodbye. Something clicked in my heart after that. I have been so down worrying about my life and my issues. Here is a man who is about to die and takes the time to share some optimistic life advice and fun with me. He is focusing on me and my life even when his is about to end. This shook me and is something I will never forget. I am so happy I met Todd and Janice even though I knew nothing about them. Meeting them has given me a will to drive forward and make the most of life. I heard a man be sentenced to death and take it on the chin. He hadn't given up, even with all that. I was worried about not being able to walk and a pain that compared to Todd's reality was insignificant. My condition was not life threatening but still I spent so much time inside my soul feeling sorry for myself and here was a man who was about to die and he has time to spread something positive into the world.

A few moments later and a porter arrived to wheel me downstairs to my appointment with Mr Quiet. When I returned, Todd's bed was empty and was being cleaned by one of the nurses. He was gone and I would not meet him again. Wherever Todd is I would like to reference another quote by Noel Coward in his memory:

"Never mind dear, we're all made the same, though some better than others."

Thank you, Todd, for taking the time to educate me with your wit, even in a time of great peril. I will do more to make this world a better place, even if it is passing on your wisdom and advice. I promise to honour a better man's advice that has lent a naive man worldwide perspective and most importantly never to be boring ever again.

There is one more story behind the curtain that I want to share with you. It came from a young man called Matt who was in his twenties and entered our ward in the middle of the night, three days into my stay. I went to sleep with an empty bed to my left following screaming man's discharge and awoke to hear a very upbeat voice chatting away to the nurses. He spoke with a familiar tone and explained to the healthcare professionals that he would be going over to the Royal Marsden later today. He had been brought into hospital by an ambulance because he was running a high fever. Then he added that he had Cancer and had been battling it for some time and knew that he could not take any medication without seeing an Oncologist first (Oncology is the study of Cancer.) He spoke with clarity and precision that I would later realise derived from experiences; this was not his first rodeo. The nurse listened to Matt and then left, presumably to call his Oncologist to get further instructions. Smokey passed the nurse post his morning commute for a smoke clutching *The Sun*. He sees Matt and offers a chirpy introduction paired with 'welcome to the madhouse' and for the first time Smokey and I agreed on something.

Matt was a burst of energy on our ward. To have someone of similar age was comforting and it was not long before he jumped out of bed and came over to sit on the stool next to my bed. As if we were back on the school playground, two boys shared stories and jokes. Having realised from his comments that Matt was living with Cancer, I did not want to pry and tried to steer away from it. We are somewhere discussing Arsenal's steady demise from 'the invincible' season and Matt starts explaining vivid details of his condition. "Seven years in total mate, the thing in my leg. Started as a golf ball and then grew to a tennis ball and before they operated on it the growth was almost the size of a football. Do you wanna see?" Matt then presented me with a slideshow of images confirming his comparisons. He has a tumour that had been growing on the top of his right leg just to the right of his crown jewels. He had documented the journey of his tumour with his iPhone. It started with a red rash and then grew to differing sphere like objects, that if I am honest looked a little like a small alien beneath his skin. His team had tried cutting it out twice alongside hours of chemotherapy. The last photo he showed me was the third resurgence of the tumour and was now the size of a small golf ball. "Luckily it wasn't in the dick" Matt blurted out. I smiled but felt awful in doing so. I am no stranger to Cancer but to sit here and laugh about returning tumours seems a little out of touch but no matter. Matt had a son and a fiancée who he was going to marry in July. Accordingly, his phone constantly pinged with colours of flowers or invitations to tasting menus which all seemed to be the same. I really enjoyed talking with Matt and hearing about his life in such detail. I admired how honest he was in not being down and out because Cancer kept kicking him, each day was a blessing and he was proof of that. The last topic of the conversation was his treatment now. Having exhausted all NHS treatments, he was now attempting to see one of the leading Cancer experts in the world. This would come at a hefty cost but given he was now being told that there was no hope for him in the NHS did he really have a choice? Matt had researched it and there was a doctor who was treating Cancer in a new way and this was his last hope. I would later face this exact conundrum of NHS vs Private. If the NHS can no longer solve your issue, then what choice do you have in reality? The truth in this question is that unless you have insurance then it is decided entirely on how much money you have making it an uneven playing field. The Cristiano Ronaldo of Cancer did not operate in the NHS, making it completely exclusive to those who can afford his time or those with enough extra income and foresight to have private medical insurance. Matt was getting married soon and I imagine that even if they were very comfortable having to pay for the two would be a struggle. I do not understand how people who are not well off get access to the best healthcare. The BBC reported that in 2016 that more than 16 million people in the UK have less than £100 saved. A hundred quid will not get you into see the specialists, it would probably cover the car parking fee though. Healthcare was not as even as the government might have you believe, and this must mean that there are a group of people in the UK suffering unnecessarily because they cannot afford private healthcare. The Guardian claims that 6% of the UK have private healthcare with the majority of these being a perk through an employer. Amongst this all I ponder which base Matt is camped in but feel too embarrassed to ask.

Our conversation was interrupted by Matt's fiancée calling with more wedding decisions. Matt shook my hand and answered the call whilst walking back to his bed and I went back to my book. The physio team came to take me off to do some leg exercises which I would compare to being as fun and running a cheese grater down ones' cheek. Upon my return to the bed of dreams, Matt was now in the corner chatting to Smokey with both laughing in unison. I loved how Matt was a burst of positive energy in the ward that normally is filled with despair. He was a man who knew this place all too well and owned it rather than being dragged down. Doctors arrived to announce Matt was off to the Royal Marsden via hospital transport. Packing up his things he was winding the nurses up claiming they had plotted to kick him out for being so talkative which made the room join in. With his backpack full he came around and shook each patients hand in the room and with that he was away for a walk.

Meeting Matt made my head spin. The reality of our conversation hit me after he left. I think he put so much effort into fighting his illness, getting married and being an all-round lovely bloke to laugh in the face of Cancer. People are so quick to wrap themselves up in problems and bathe in it. The man with the smile, bald head and tennis ball tumour was not going to let the killer disease get one over on him and I hugely admired his determination to continue life with a smile. I thought how shallow I had been worrying about not being able to walk for a week and living in hospital. Todd had walked tall in the face of death and Matt inspired me to buck up and see the Brightside. The lives that I came into contact within hospital have changed me for good and although I could not see it at the time it gave me perspective I was in urgent need for.

Just after dinner, Smokey wheeled over waxing lyrical about Matt. This was the first time I had engaged with him one on one. He told me that when they had spoken Smokey had been honest about how down and out he was. Matt parted with him by slipping a tenner into Smokey's palm followed by "I've been where you are and hope this helps." This sentiment engulfed me, and I replied with "what a lovely bloke" knowing that no words I knew could articulate the man I'd met well enough.

Drugs

The pain team visited me on my third day to discuss the best options for getting me comfortable whilst I waited to see Mr Quiet. The best option available to me was to take the medicine they recommended which would keep my pain under control. Alongside this process I was to work with the Physio team on using my frame and crutches to improve my mobility. This was a peculiar lesson for me as I was learning how to mobile as if nothing further would be done. The concept of being trapped in this state permanently is one that leered over my head constantly as I considered that if this is never fixed, walking with aids will become my life's work. I used this to spur me on and accept anything that was offered to me to see the bright side of life.

The drugs are given to you by the nurses, or with a gentle reminder if they are super busy. Smokey never noticed what time it was or when drugs were due. He would always follow any request I asked with his own interjection of "any drugs for me nurse?" He would also play a game of confusing nurses in telling lies about when he was due his next fix. For example, Smokey would be given a drug he gets three times a day (normally aligned after each meal.) Around an hour after breakfast he would request another painkiller claiming he had not received it. The nurse would then check the chart and remind him he had been given it forty minutes previously. To this he would act confused and out of sync pretending that the situation he found himself in which the nurses would play along with. I believed this act for the first few times he performed it, but then noticed he did this every day to try and get an extra pain killer into his body. The nurses would never give him one without checking the chart and this meant he never succeeded in his deceptive plot. What made me laugh was that he would continue to do so without changing the routine. I never knew whether this was to pass the time or just to get the most he could whilst being there. Either way the man had a performative ability that was annoyingly watchable.

The drugs I took were addictive which they don't tell you at the time. If you take opiate pain killers for long enough your body will latch onto them and yearn for them physically as if your brain needs them for bodily function. If you were to suddenly stop taking them, you would get withdrawal sickness which has a large list of nasty side effects. At the time when you are in pain, drugs are amazing because they give you a break. When the agony is silenced it can provide a calm that is worth its weight in gold. The issue is that the medicine does not just take the pain away, it does lots of other things to the body. I was on over ten different drugs with a plethora of side effects in all areas. I needed the drugs because I had bulges on my spine that were compressing nerves which run down to my left leg. A fundamental problem (or challenge as my Father would say) was that the pain team clearly explained that nerve pain is very difficult to treat and, in some cases,, it was impossible to remove the pain altogether even if they were using the strongest drugs possible. They started me on Pregabalin which was to help with the nerve compression, but this would only work in 7-10 days. The Oxycodone was for the treatment of severe pain and literally puts you off your face. The drugs I took also made going to the bathroom for a number two impossible so to wash every meal down I took orange flavour laxatives. My life was nothing if not graceful.

The pain team would visit me every few days to check in on how I was doing. Each time they would come and each time I would still be hurting. They would tweak my drugs so that my chart looked like it had been handled by a toddler. It would work by the Pain team requesting the drugs and that would prompt the pharmacist to come the following morning with a special delivery and set you up. I always enjoyed chatting to the pharmacist as they had the inside scoop on all the drugs and what they did. I was shocked to read some of the side effects and thought how many people just happily take what the doctor gives them without thinking about it? It is not a criticism but, in a world, where we question everything from fake news to our democratic leaders why do we have such blind faith in drugs because they are administered by a Doctor?

Despite all my complaining, the worst side effect for me, and I am sure for most people, is constipation. This is all part of a viscous cycle that I found myself drowning in. You are made to eat three square meals a day, there is no way to avoid this for obvious reasons. The drugs dry up your intestines which in turn dries the faeces in your bowel causing a blockage. This leaves you sitting in bed most days feeling as you have destroyed two pizzas form Dominos (you don't normally order two, but it was Tuesday and you got an extra one for free, we've all been there!) After the bloated feeling comes the sweats and clammy hands. Then enter the headache and feeling very odd indeed and this can be a serious problem. Each meal is followed by the laxative powder which tastes like dirty dish water. Level two is having a thick syrup which is very similar to a mouldy cough syrup. Whilst you are taking these you enter a constant discourse about your toilet activities with every nurse you speak to. Like the weather in real life, poo is a common conversation inside a hospital. "When was the last time you went?" is normally how it is presented, and you talk about it without naming it. Delicate wordplay by the nurses avoid embarrassment but when the syrups and powders don't work then you move to a whole new level of awkwardness.

On one morning, I woke up and felt about ten stone heavier. I had sweated so much in the night that my bed sheet was wet, and clothes stuck to me like glue. When Sarah checked in and asked me how I was, I quickly complained. She checked me over and asked the usual soft questions, to which I did not have a good reply "3 and a half days." I knew what would follow but it still surprises you. Sarah told me an enema might be a good idea because if we leave it, I will get sicker and on top of all my issues we could do with as little drama as possible. She added that if I drank a few litres of Prune juice this could also do the job. Failing this the nurses would insert a fluid into my back passage which when in, breaks down any solid matter and then rushes back out.

Prune juice did nothing and my reward would be given at seven PM that evening. The nurses came in a pair as given NHS protocol you must have someone supervise you when it is more 'intimate.' As the deed was being done and I will leave out the details, I could not help but think that every other man in this ward is now listening to me having liquid squirted into my ass. Looking back, I would be embarrassed or ashamed, but the truth is at the time you just don't care. When you're in hospital you are in such a state that it all blows over you. I say that, and it isn't exactly true, but you get where I am going. The nurse was finished and blurted out the final instruction "hold it in for about twenty minutes and then go to the bathroom." I can share with you that those twenty minutes felt like a two hundred and I must have looked like a blue whale slowly dying on a beach as I twisted and turned trying to keep all the liquid inside. I think I held out for seventeen and good morning Mr President! I felt better after that but three days later I was in the same position and I endured a few more which never got any better. I felt so low not even being able to perform the most basic of human tasks, lying in that bed you feel useless and a waste of human being. Telling you that is to reveal that people in those situations are far from a waste of space and in truth are probably so drugged up they would not know whether they were coming or going, they just need a little help.

The side effects I have experienced are: Headaches, nausea, hallucinations, constipation, shaking, sweats, passing blood, internal aches and pains, suicidal/depressing thoughts, weight gain and states of confusion to name but a few. The drugs can take you out of your mind without you having any idea that your behaviour has switched. In my case, I had a day when I had convinced myself the Doctors were plotting against me because the pain was not easing. I spent the afternoon writing on a scrap of paper all the reasons why the doctors would have it in for me. After making my hysterical list I then settled on the escape plan of self-discharge after rounds the next day and simply crutching myself out the front door. I cannot tell you how ludicrous all of this was. I made it all worse by telling my partner's mother my elaborate scheme and she did an amazing task of realising I was not of sound mind and gently brought me back to earth. This took nearly an hour, but after much discussion and an objective explanation I was settled that I was not a victim of the next Harold Shipman. Writing this all down is laughable now, but I can tell you it was all real in my head. The drugs that flowed in my blood had taken my mind outside itself and had it not been for other's help I may well have tried to leave my ward and had all manner of nasty consequences arrive in my life. You have no idea that you are on another planet and the sheer power of these tablets demands respect.

Dealing with the drugs has been an ongoing journey but one that I would recommend you don't do alone. The best advice I have for this scenario is be open and honest with those around you. Telling the nurse, I went to bed with thoughts of not wanting to be here anymore (which is scary enough) is not easy. But upon chatting it through, I can understand that it's not Craig thinking in that darkness but the chemicals pumping through my body. Speaking up about all the changes in your body can make a huge difference, so ask questions and understand what you are taking because understanding why it's dark around you can sometimes let in some sunshine.

Quiet Please

The first days in hospital had been a shock to my system. I had a huge amount of time on my hands which I tried to fill by putting positive energy into my current challenge. Focusing on my Father's optimism I wanted to find out a little more about the surgical procedure in detail. This was done in a Louis Lane style of interviewing nurses who had treated people like me. I also spoke to the ward's trauma expert. Rupert came to my bed and introduced himself with a smile and a mouthful of jokes. He asked if I knew the actual science of what was going on in my back and if surgery was the next step, what that would entail? Shaking my head confirmed that my CC in double award science GCSE would not help me here which prompted Rupert to whip out his phone. Scrolling through YouTube he showed me a digital video of what the procedure would involve. Seeing a computer-generated version of the spine is much easier to cope with and the simple format even meant sense to me. In simple terms: they would cut through three layers of muscle and once at my vertebrate remove the bulges with a chop and then close me up. Simple enough I thought.

Anyone that has had surgery will know that anxiety is perfectly normal. For me, seeing the images in the video helped me accept that this was a simple operation. I would also like to add that going onto YouTube can lead you down the rabbit hole. My advice to you is: DO NOT WATCH THE ACTUAL SURGERY VIDEO as this is much more harrowing. Rupert gave me this advice which fulfilling my masculinity, I ignored and watched after he left. Seventeen seconds in I was seeing the human spine, and this was very troubling. I quickly exited it and did not revisit the subject matter.

So much had happened since my diagnosis that I had forgotten surgery was not yet confirmed. I was to see Mr Quiet (a spinal surgeon) 6 days into my hospital stay. He would be the one who would ultimately decide the next steps. Having done my research, I had discovered he also had worked privately at a local clinic. The predicted wait times on the NHS were very long and given that I was not dying, this could take a while. The day before I met with Mr Quiet, I spoke with my father on this topic. I knew that given the ridiculous cost of spinal surgery I could never ask someone to fund it. I did not have thousands of pounds at my disposal so I could not pay for it myself. I presented my findings to my Dad over the phone in as much detail as possible and then just left them to take it all in. I was aware that given the severity of my condition I would not be able to walk or leave bed until I had the surgery or some other resolution. Whatever waiting time, these things are sent to test us and the only is up, right?

An hour before I was to meet Mr Quiet, Dad called me. He calmly told me that I had their full support and whatever the cost, if the wait was ridiculous, I had permission to entertain the private option which my Father and Stepmother would pay for. Hearing those words filled my empty heart with emotion. Dad has done so much for me through being a single parent and everything in-between. My sister and I never went without and he had supported me through every dream I had. He was retired with no income but just told me he would find a way if I needed it and this would change our relationship forever. Alongside this his wife would happily put up half the money to a son who is not her own, but she would love just the same.

My lift arrived by way of hospital porter with a wheelchair. I had not sat in a chair for nearly a week and starred at my nemesis with focused eyes. The problem with sitting was that it required my left thigh to be in contact with the chair and have downward pressure on the nerves that are still extremely tender. I did not want to make a fuss, so I rolled out of bed and sat down hoping for the best outcome.

There is popular game amongst children which has seen precedence on social media named 'the floor is lava.' If you know this activity you might be able to picture my journey to see Mr Quiet, my bum being the feet and the wheelchair being hot and painful lava. Down two floors and attempting to make small talk with the porter as a distraction, I immediately regretted not taking a pain killer before setting off on my quest across middle earth. Enter a packed waiting room of people who do not live in hospital and I am turning some heads. I am wriggling as if a small squirrel has entered my tracksuit bottoms and gasping in pain. The porter parks me near the wall and all eyes are on the twitching man who cannot get comfortable. A nurse comes over and asks me if I am ok, I explain I am here to see Mr Quiet. My appointment was in twenty minutes so the nurse offered me a glass of water, I was not thirsty but accepted to be polite. I was going out of my mind. Sitting down was now impossible so I was leaning against the wheelchair which did not have breaks on, using the wall as support. The nurse returned with a cup of water, I took one sip and then dropped the cup as my back started to spasm uncontrollably. Realising that I was now the most popular attraction at the fair and that my pain was drifting out of control the nurse slipped away to see if Mr Quiet could see me now rather than on the hour. Lucky for me and unlucky for the voyeurs in the crowd, Mr Quiet was free, and my time had come to meet the man behind the legend.

Mr Quiet is a man of very few words. He greeted me in and we shook hands in a soft embrace as the nurse parked me next to his desk. I could see my MRI scan on his computer screen in a small and dingy office. He then asked me to stand up so he could asses me physically. Using the chair frame as a pivot, I got to my feet realising this was not the time to complain. I have always had a huge respect for doctors as if they are on another plain altogether. The knowledge, skill and temperament required to be a doctor is immense, and to be a have been a spinal surgeon for thirty years is beyond my small mind's comprehension. Whatever Quiet wanted he would get from my frail body.

Standing with as much balance as a new-born lamb, I bit my lip in pain. "Please could you take a few steps for me attempting to evenly distribute the pressure through both feet if possible." I put my left foot forward and the weight was too much for my body to handle, I fell forward and caught myself the edge of the wheelchair. As my calamity was unfolding Mr Quiet's eyes were on me like a hawk scanning his prey. I got back up slowly and then he wanted to see me bend forward. I tried three times and could only manage a pathetic few degrees which was followed by an invitation to take a seat as the analysis was over, which was wonderful news to my forehead which was dripping with sweat.

I was then to get the most detailed and precise presentation of my condition to date. Using the scan as reference Quiet laid out my options as I had heard before. In his opinion surgery was the only thing that would solve my problems and he was confident that he was up to the task. Now it was time for the million-dollar question – "At least twelve weeks but could be much longer." Three months to be bed bound, loaded on drugs and unable to walk seemed impossible to achieve so I asked him what options there were privately? "I could get you booked in for the start or May" which was in three and a half weeks' time. "It will cost around £7000 for the operation and the aftercare. You would be in hospital for one might and it would take your body 4-6 weeks to recover all being well (massive understatement.) This procedure comes with an 80-90% success rate. It also comes with a 4% chance that you will lose the ability to walk or control of your bladder and bowels permanently."

In my eyes those were good odds. They would enable me to hopefully tackle the pain in my body and move forward with my life. At this stage my mind was obsessed and plagued with my condition. I ignored friends on my phone and was slowly disappearing into myself. Agony pulsated through my veins engulfing my heart, mind and soul. My optimistic outlook on life was shot and being run over by a Land Rover. I no longer took pleasure in jokes and if looking at a glass to determine if it was half full or half empty, I would simply pick up the glass and smash it against the wall. I nodded and agreed to what Mr Quiet had offered. He informed me that the administration department would be in touch with me to confirm the details but all being well my spine would be on his operating table very soon.

Once back home in my ward, I called my father and just started crying uncontrollably. News of the surgery was a good thing, but it was overwhelming. He kept me upbeat as ever and agreed once the paperwork was sent over, he would come across country to fill it all out with me. This was a minor operation in the scheme of the body but contemplating a blade cutting your back open is tough to comprehend. Scared and sitting in my hospital bed I imagined waking up and never being to walk or use the toilet. I dwelled on all the worst-case scenarios because I was on my way to giving up, even though the solution was right in front of me. I was tumbling down a well and unlike Batman, it was unclear if I would ever make it out.

The following morning, I was contacted by the administration team of the private hospital about seven miles away. There were two things that needed to happen before my operation could be confirmed:

1. Full payment of £7000 received seven days before the date of the procedure.

2. I must attend a pre-assessment at the hospital to screen or infections.

I had assumed that one could pay a sum as large as my fee in instalments, this was wrong and there was no room for negotiation regarding this. Wanting to make it as simple for my father as possible I tried to barter but the voice on the phone was playing hardball. In regard to my check, I politely explained that I was living in hospital and if the tests could be provided here? This question was smacked around the chops with hostility and venom thus highlighting our favourite boxing match of Public vs. Private. The voice bluntly educated me that NHS hospitals do not screen for the infections they do almost in a tone of establishment hysteria and insisted firmly that I must be at their hospital in person or else. I could not walk or sit down so travelling in a car was hard for me to imagine but this mattered not. They know you're desperate so they know you will figure it out. No emotion or empathy, this was business. I was defeated and chose a date with no idea how I would get there or what state my body would be in when I arrived.

The evening before I was due to go to my pre assessment the pain team visited me. They refused to let me get into a regular car due to my own safety and requested a hospital transport which would take me there and bring me back. This was a surprise as I had been constantly aware that the two healthcare systems did no favours for the other side. The private hospital had offered a ride service from them at a cost of a few hundred pounds which I laughed down the phone when I was told the price so to the NHS were again going the extra mile, or so I thought. Ninety minutes before I was due at the private hospital, a nurse told me that I would not be getting a lift because the policy dictated that it could only be between NHS hospitals and not to private ones. They also offered me an ambulance service at the cost of over a hundred pounds. Given the late notice they asked me to cancel my appointment (which would cancel my potential operation) and reschedule. At this point I went full Queen of Hearts and just exploded in fury inside but being English just thanked the nurse for giving me the worst possible news. I knew my Dad would have been there to take me but because he lived 150 miles away there was not enough time to get here and get me there on time. With my only option left to me was to call my partners mother and beg for a lift under very short time pressure. For reasons beyond me, Jane came to the rescue and said she would bring the car which would flatten down and get me to where I needed to be. Predicting this was going to be as fun as dragging naked feet over smashed glass I asked the nurse if I could take a pain killer now and also have an emergency one in case, we saw a repeat of twitching Craig. I think the team on the ward realised they had shafted me so against the normal strict medication rules my request was granted and an extra pill was given for the road.

I was angry, upset and vulnerable. With a backpack over my right shoulder I crutched to the front entrance by myself. Getting there with ten minutes to spare which was much needed wiping down time as my face glistened with sweat. In all of my hospital time it is astounding how quickly the body starts to break down. As I leaned against the wall waiting for my lift, I watched people coming and going out of the hospital's main entrance. Patients, visitors and staff all on feet showing a variety of people from all walks of life. I stared in envy as they all seemed so carefree. I could not remember the last time I did something for me on my own that was not related to my health problems. In that moment I began to see an inch of happiness in my sky. Being inside a hospital ward can flood you with doubt and breathing in fresh air and a blue sky was as potent to my soul as the morphine that induced my pain. I considered how self-centred I had become and in this I had totally written off everything else going on around me. A few moments after my philosophical plights, my knight in shining armour arrived. The journey was crap but we won't dwell on that. By the time I got to the hospital I was knackered and my t-shirt was sodden. When shown the waiting room I just put all my weight against the wall in exhaustion. The nurse (in a super posh uniform) called me in and then offered me a seat. I just made my way over the bed and slumped over rasping with deep breaths. "Are you OK Craig?" She gently asked. "I made it" I replied and with that my face lit up with a smile. One more level closer to the final boss stage and nothing was going to stop me now.

The Last Unicorn

After my big day off I felt nothing like Ferris Bueller. I made it back to the hospital and flopped back onto my familiar bed with the grace of a walrus on an iceberg. Ten days in and surgery was now confirmed at the private hospital, all I had to do was get through the next few weeks. When you are in an NHS hospital, there is always something going on, it is a pond brimming with life. Take the morning after my day trip, Smokey woke up in a particularly buoyant mood. He was receiving a haircut and a shave from one of the nurse students who had promised it if he was still here by this date. The student arrived on morning rounds with Smokey waving a Gillette Razor in the air as if it was the winning lottery ticket "I cannot wait for my tidy up, I've been waiting for this" (yes, it sounded as creepy as it reads.) Sat down in a chair, the patient had his head shaved bald, and the same method was applied to his face. Like a snooker ball, Smokey's head now shone like one of the moons in orbit of our planet. His face was a light with joy and it reminded me that in here the simplest of things can give one satisfaction. Smokey was still drinking at night but was still evading campus patrol. When he was on the phone to his friends, he would ask for a list of items mixed with a bizarre word. "Can you bring me some deodorant, toothpaste, Mars Bars and a green rug" would be an example. Given my limited ability in deduction I could only assume this was code for contraband. They were very sneaky about it though, as I watched for a passing of cargo and I was always bitterly disappointed. However, they were doing it, booze was on my ward on a regular basis but for now Smokey was sober and looking trim thanks to his fresh cut.

When the young nurse made it to my bed, she offered me the same treatment. I laughed this off as at twenty nine I still had the stubble of a babies bottom, and to try and cut my Russel Brand hair would maybe be a task too big for one person. We laughed and chatted about trivial topics from the outside world. I was also a hot topic of conversation on the ward as with my appointment going well and surgery being confirmed, crippled Craig may soon be exiting. The student's I had looking after me were all exceptional. To think I spent my university years sipping cheap snake bite and waddling around a hockey pitch made me embarrassed when a second-year nurse was fully immersed in all aspects of my care. They could offer insight into things the Doctor's never went into such as the truth about side effects or why it was important to have an injection in your stomach daily to stop blood clots. They were smart, compassionate and always cheered me up.

That same morning saw the arrival of a new patient in Screaming man and Matt's old bed (the one to my left.) His name was Tom and he was another highflyer. Owner of his own business in the local area clad with laptop, tablet and multiple mobile phones, he had that professional aurora. Tom was here to have a crack in his hip fixed. He had damaged the bone with a fall and tomorrow he was due to go under the knife in my hospital. Throwing himself into ward life he asked me for my story which by now I had perfected into a few short sentences but as I performed my lines his face seemed to light up with interest and that was because his daughter had my exact condition and had been living with it for six years. This revelation launched us into the gritty details of comparing each other's notes. I was slightly worse off being I could not walk or sit, and she had never been hospitalised by it. She did however have to leave university because of the pain/drug balance which threw her life a little off course. Two spinal injections and a pain management group meeting that she attended regularly, and her spinal issues had dictated most all of her life to date. Whilst listening to the story, I kept thinking if this was so bad and had been in her body for so long, then why was Surgery not an option? The answer to this was: Fear.

Tom's daughter did not want to engage with Spinal surgery because the thought of it was terrifying. This simple explanation meant that every avenue would be tried before laying down on the table and being cut open. The story did offer me a strange comfort as she had tried all the things I had been offered as less invasive measures and they had failed. When going straight for surgery I pondered if it was just the dramatic side of me wanting the most extreme solution rather than taking the logical conservative options first. I can be quite honest now that if I had to live with how I was in that hospital for six years, I would have more likely tried to throw myself off the roof than walk amongst apologetic passive treatment plans. It sounds crazy, but there is no way I would let my fear stop my surgery, even though this conversation was ringing alarm bells, what the hell did I really know about this procedure and the risks? Had I made a rash decision and acted on the pain rather than the sensible explanation. Chatting this out with Tom made me realise that one thing you should never do is compare, especially with health. Every human body is different and just because we both have bulges on our discs, does not mean we understand the yin to each other's yang. The truth was that my body had removed the element of choice from my heart. I was stuck in bed unable to do anything but conjure drug fuelled stories. Whilst Tom's daughter limped but could walk and had now taken drugs for so long, they were ineffective. I longed to meet her and talk to someone who understood exactly what I was feeling. Just before dinner Tom's wife and daughter would visit and I would learn much more about this family.

When Mary entered our room, I knew she was Tom's daughter immediately. The movement of her body across the hospital floor sung to me and I knew that this young woman was dealing with serious back troubles. Mary was shy when her father introduced me. She did not seem very interested in having a conversation but humoured her parental initiation to do so. Sensing the awkwardness, I launched into my life story about my back. Mary was polite and listened quietly and then when I had finished, she set out her six years of suffering. The drugs had done so much to change her she now attended a support group which focuses on severe pain management without medication. She admitted she was miserable, had gained weight, lost her university ambitions amongst a life of a pain you don't understand unless you have it. Mary was a fighter and was going to put her body on the line to do what she needed to do. Surgery was not an option for her and I respected the bravery it took to make that choice. In hospital you are mostly surrounded by people who have had the choice over their treatment taken away due to events spiralling out of control. These wards are not filled with people who are taking small and passive steps to manage moments of the mundane in a hurricane of agony. Everyone has their own path to tread and as much as Mary's parents wanted the surgery that was not their call. Mary and me were also very lucky to have the support of people in our family willing to help us. My conversation ended when Mary's brothers arrived, and the magical blue curtain was drawn. I thanked her for the company and wished her luck. She said nothing but nodded as if to agree with me. That connection gave me a little lift as I realised in a sea of troubles I was swimming in, I was not the only one adrift.

The next morning and Tom was on the water and food ban that all people who are having general aesthetic endure. The nurses were cleaning him all over with disinfecting wipes and making sure when the call came, he was good to go. Surgery for something that is not urgent works a little like the meat counter in Sainsburys. You pull a ticket and based on what number they are on now and the queue in front of the glass you make a suitable guess on your waiting time. Hospital adds the fact there are people who are in desperate need for rib eye or pork belly and therefore can get a later number but be seen first. I don't think anyone can criticise this process, but it can make the pause before the operation long. Tom waited the whole day and was told mid-afternoon that he would not be operated on. He was upbeat and quickly requested a sandwich and a cup of tea to restore him.

Smokey was busy that morning as well. He had received a visit from the discharge team who arrived with news that he must leave hospital because he was now stable. He was on a ward for acute patients and his bed was in extremely high demand. As soon as the sentence sprinted into the air, Smokey erupted in a flourish of agony and despair. He started to roll across his bed claiming that his ankle was throbbing in sharp flashes of pain. "Sleep is impossible because of how uncomfortable I am" he protested, but that could be that he spends the evenings on the piss. He then moves onto complaint of his wrist that has shooting throbs and he is not even smoking anymore and just surviving on nicotine patches (I have witnessed him wheel outside at least three times so far today.) Lastly, he claims that his mental health is spiralling out of control and if taken to the outside world he would almost certainly end up hurting himself. The discharge team listen intently. The words that they must come across most days from those who find the hospital ward a comforting home and something worth fighting for. They thank Smokey for his honesty and promise to return soon with some news.

No news is good news and Smokey was no different. As wise ward dwellers we know that nothing major happens after five. This is because the bosses have gone home and the NHS is based on a tower of dotted lines requiring the golden signatures. No discharge would be processed, not until tomorrow morning. Success had created hunger. As dinner arrived Smokey refused it as he was going to order himself a Chinese takeaway. Thirty minutes later he wheeled himself down 2 floors and across the hospital on his Zimmer with his 'painful ankle and throbbing wrist' and collected a bag of MSG soaked goodies. He passes the nurse bay and throws a bag of prawn crackers to them as thanks. Smokey gets in his bed and devours his order and looks like the cat who got the cream.

It would be three more days before Tom would be taken for his operation. The emergency department was keeping the general surgeons extremely busy. Each day they prepped and starved him and each day he would be relieved that it was not going to happen. Tom was very polite about it, but I could see it grate even the calmest of temperaments. After his operation he was home the next day which was not strictly kosher with the surgeon, but I think the ward sister was happy to have the bed. When he left, Mary was there supporting her father the best she could dressed in sad eyes that met mine with empathy. Then, like that, my neighbour was gone and to be filled with many more men. I would never connect with another bed buddy like I did Todd, Matt & Tom. They all gave me so much in perspective, faith and friendship. Sick men provided me with a renewed faith in human beings, if shadows can be smiled at in this ward then everything else must be a breeze. Connections kept me sane in a time of madness. As I am deep within the avenues of contemplation, I am looking at the bed being wiped by a nurse whilst Smokey is wheeling in wielding a takeaway Pizza and climbing into back into bed. "Ham and Pineapple?" I asked. "Meat Feast brother" he replied.

Pride

"A man's pride can be his downfall, and he needs to learn when to turn to others for support and guidance."

The worst thing about Sciatica is the inability to do anything for yourself. You cannot walk, sit, bend down, stretch up and all other physical activities that are required to get one through the day. My day is much simpler than it normally is, but even raising the top of the bed up so I can eat my food without choking causes me serious pain. I am rubbish in asking for help. This comes from being independent Craig, who is active, impulsive and hyper. I love throwing myself headfirst into life which in turn is why I have made so many mistakes. It is also why I can do well in scenarios others struggle. I was confident in groups and the first to get involved. This sometimes landed me in trouble... who am I kidding? It always landed me in trouble but at least I got Involved. Well I did, until now.

Considering how much I have shared so far I will take you back to my first morning waking up in hospital where a young student nurse came over to ask "would like a shower or a bed wash Craig?" This could not have been a bigger inquiry and was one that filled me with dread. A bed wash is where the nurse has a bowl of water and gently flannels your body with warm water whilst you lay there and take it. They remove your clothing (behind everyone's favourite curtain) and just soap you down. I could sense my inner voice squirming with embarrassment at the thought of this action. The whole idea of this was odd. I had images of a corpse in a funeral parlour that is just a lump of cold meat being dressed up for their final party and was in no mood to live out this fantasy just yet.

The shower was the next option. I love showers and need them every day in the real world. If I don't wash, I get fidgety and grumpy and feel like a grubby pig. So whatever it took, I was washing that morning. The nurse carried my washing materials and clean clothes in a sick basin (which had not been used for its initial purpose) and shadowed me over to the bathroom at the entrance to our ward. The shower had rails to hold onto and I was determined. I got to shower room and the nurse was placing the towel on the side just as I attempted to grab the rail to steady myself I missed it and went crashing into the wall. I screamed in pain and felt my back go into spasm. (Back spasms feel like there are small animals in your back with little balls. They are then squeezing, throwing and biting these balls. It hurts like hell and leaves me frozen in state of statue like stillness until it passes. I hate them because they literally cripple me completely.) My eyes were welling up with tears. This was unbearable. The nurse helped me to lean against the wall and held my hand until the spasm played out. It stopped and I drew a sharp breath. Then the question came "would you like me to help you shower?" This nurse was barely over 20. At least half my size and a student doing her training. I was embarrassed and vulnerable. I was still adamant I could do these basic human tasks and declined her help on the basis of stroking my pathetic ego. I should have said yes and accepted the gesture of kindness but my stupid pride kicked in with all these thoughts exploding in my head:

1. It is inappropriate for another woman to see me naked?
2. I am strong enough to shower alone. I don't need her help!
3. Am I cheating on my girlfriend?
4. She will judge my body.
5. She will think I am fat and ugly!
6. She will tell her colleagues how fat and ugly this crippled man is.
7. I can't do this – any of this. Ask for help Craig.
8. Accepting help makes you weak – Buck up!
9. Just give up.
10. Don't wash. Lie in filth. Bathe in pity.
11. Close your eyes and never open them again.

I could have asked for a male nurse. I could have asked for time to recover from the spasm and I could have just not showered. I ignored all of these sensible thoughts and replied "No thank you. I'll be fine." She asked again. I refused. She could read every thought on my face and I was going bright red, riddled with shame. I was stubborn, too proud and idiotic to ask for help. She left and I attempted to shower alone. The effort was useless as I couldn't use my arms, bend or use washing gel. I leant against the wall clinging to the hot water and just let it flow over me, washing my shame away. In that moment I have never felt as worthless in my life. All I could focus on was my pain and misery and nothing else apart from a compelling self-hatred of what I had become.

This cycle of destructive behaviour continued with anything that was slightly embarrassing. I hated the fact I couldn't do it by myself and I suffered through horrific pain just because of pride. A few days after the first wash I slipped in the shower and banged my head against the wall. Laying on the bathroom floor my head was pounding, and the room seemed a little fuzzy. I was then overcome with fear as I had no idea how I would get back to my feet. Ignoring the red emergency cord, the next closest aid was the toilet bowl. Hooking my elbow against the rim I lifted my broken body off the floor. This took several attempts which included a slip and dive into the toilet water which just made me laugh. I figure the lavatories in hospital must be cleaner than most, so all was not bad. Halfway up and I take a breather on the loo seat as my lungs recover and my head continues to pound. I had a headache for the rest of the day, a slight bump on my head and didn't shower for the following two days for fear of another slip. Not once did I consider asking for any assistance. This was because the washing was my only independent outlet being on my own, naked and cleaning myself. If I had given that up, then everything in my life was done by other people. All of this made sense at the time, crystal clear like the toilet water that kissed my hand.

I learned a lot from that experience. Pride can be such a crippling vice on your sensible thought process. When you are in pain and unable to do things it's hard to ask for help even when you are desperate for it. Overcoming it is a journey but in my case the actions of being showered or being assisted taking medicine is something these healthcare professionals do every day. It's their job to help people get better and to cope with the pain they are in. They don't judge and are lovely about it. Having accepted their help on many awkward moments they respect your pride, humanity and make it almost bearable (almost.)

In my last week in the NHS hospital when the black dog was permanently laying on the foot of my bed, Shower nurse came over and caught me off guard. "You're becoming part of the family, now aren't you?" I was confused by this sentence and queried it. "It is just you have been here so long; you have become one of us." This made me cry and in trying to spit a word out my hand was cradled and squeezed gently. She smiled at me and just held my hand whilst I kept apologising. I think this moment hit me hard because I realised how stupid I had been in the shower having not respected this young woman who had a kindness that could light up the bleakest of rooms. Shower nurse could now read my mind and we had an open conversation which was dominated by me praising her. This human moment will stay with me for a long time and is something that when we struggle people can always surprise you when you ask for help. If this twenty-year-old was to remain in the NHS, I cannot fathom how many people she will save just as she did me and I am forever grateful for everything she did.

I think in my life I hold a huge amount of pointless pride. When I am pain free, I chose to do things on my own because I think I know best. The truth is I don't and could gain much more from others. I have lost my job because of the condition and once I was free of hospitals, I would be starting from zero. Once you have tasted toilet water everything else after is just champagne.

Pride comes before the fall – Literally, I fell over in the shower and it fucking hurt.

Be smart: Ask for help.

Nurses

It is very rare in this life to come across selfless acts of kindness. When one encounters them, it gives a moment of relief, peace, or a beat of silence. These are to be appreciated and treasured. Providing such a gift is the essence of a nurse's job 12 hours a day.

I lived in the NHS hospital for just over three and a half weeks. I met a variety of nurses who cared for me around the clock. They work in shifts of 12 hours (8-8 normally but others do shorter days.) You have the Ward sisters, Sisters, nurses, nursing assistants and nursing students and you can determine this based on what uniform they wear. They distribute your drugs at the correct times. They do your regular observations. They listen to every word you say with a keen intent. They understand your condition and hold a wealth of knowledge. They are the heart and soul of the hospital and keep it ticking, beat by beat.

Nurses are the only constant in the NHS hospital. They are always there, and a simple press of your bed alarm will have one in front of you in moments. They run the wards, assist the doctors, offer kindness, shave and wash you (if you'll let them) and even feed you if you so desire. In my experience there is nothing they would not do to help you be more comfortable. I met so many nurses and singling out any of them seems unfair, but these few examples represent to me what they are all about. I could have filled this entire book with examples, but that has been done by many a greater voice, so I hope these anecdotes share a piece of my gratitude.

Nurse Navy was sitting in the corner of the ward doing her notes on our charts around eleven am on my fifth morning inside. I was reading my John Grisham thriller pretending I understood the legal jargon when Doctor mean entered. Without any explanation he announced, "The Physio's have cleared you and it is time for you to be discharged." This was a very confusing sentence and one that sent me into a panic. My pain was not under control at this point and it was before my surgery was confirmed in the infancy of my stay. He offered no explanation and flicked his way through my chart in a flippant manner. I was stunned into silence and had no idea what the reason behind this assault was. The doctor then started talking to the nurse about my condition and the details of my case. Nurse Navy seemed confused as she did not have these on the tip of her tongue. The doctor who was unsatisfied left the nurse and me without any more discussion. I started to breathe deeply and panic. I was not able to walk and the pain was out of control. The thought of going home and being away from constant care sent my head into a spin and one where I lost myself. I was now hyper ventilating and almost deep into a panic attack when Nurse Navy launched onto my bed, got me to sit up and control my breath taking through showing me the slow inhale and exhale techniques. In and out, slowly slowly catch a monkey and I was coming around. When relaxed on my bed I had a million questions which I was now rapidly firing at Navy. If I was going home was, I going to get a carer to my house or how would it work with me being crippled and unable to perform basic tasks? Nurse Navy listening intently and then explained she would get the Senior Sister of the ward who would be able to answer all of my questions. Moments later The Boss Sister was by my bed side. She explained that what the doctor had meant to say but didn't, was that the Physio team had said I was safe to go home from their team's perspective. They had assessed me on the crutches and frames and were happy with how I was moving but this was only one of the infinity stones. I was under several departments. For me to be released I needed all of their sign off and that was not happening today. This was a logical explanation and I was now curious as to why it was not explained to me like this by the doctor. The Boss Sister explained the time pressure doctors are under etc but I was pissed off. I requested that I have another doctor and had no interest in his apology (classic pride strikes again) and that was the end of that. This whole situation did not need to occur if the doctor had explained and taken a moment longer in engaging with me, the patient. The care of nurse navy to calm me in a stressful scenario was brilliantly supported by her superior coming in and resolving it. All that it took was simple communication and in a flash of smoke I never saw Doctor Mean again.

The nurses at night were a smaller team but were often busy when things livened up. An evening regular, Rachel, had recently qualified and by chance went to primary school with my partner and picked this up after recognising her when she had visited me. This little connection to the outside world gave me a comforting feeling when chatting with her. Before lights out she would often wheel in the night trolley of drugs followed by a request for late night snacks. This would comprise of the sandwiches and biscuits left over from lunch. On occasion, a midnight snack would be a dream and Smokey would often request three or four to add to his tuck cupboard. It must sound stupid, but these little acts of generosity are such rush of sunlight in your heart when stuck in bed night and day that it is always appreciated. Rachel also had the rare ability of talking to you as if you were in a pub or on a bus or even at home. She never dwelled on medical chat or points to do with hospitals or conditions, instead she loved a chin wag about anything and anyone. One of her main grumbles about work was about 'Granny Time.' This is where a family with a sick elderly relative brings the OAP into hospital claiming their condition has worsened and must be admitted urgently. This is of course fine, and they normally are admitted but this coincidently coincides with the family going on holiday. This is a big trend in the NHS according to Rachel. So, if you are planning a trip to the Algarve please make sure Nana is well tended to and not in hospital because it is cheaper than a care home.

One dark and dank evening I was struggling with the enormity of my condition and the severity of spinal surgery. Unable to sleep due to the anxiety, I was crying in a ball on my bed at around 2am. Everyone was asleep on my ward (even Smokey) and without me realising a hand lay gently on my shoulder. The first words I spoke were "I don't want to be here anymore." The nurse walked round and bent down, so we were eye to eye. She simply said, "That's OK but can you tell me why?" What followed was a heartfelt monologue of emotion explaining my fears, loneliness and desire to disappear. She did not judge but instead listened to me speak through my dribbling snot and cold streams of tears. After I had emptied my soul, she started to offer solutions to all my questions. Most importantly she reminded me that one of the drugs I am taking can cause deep depression and suicidal thoughts which might marry with the darkness radiating my head. This does not mean that all I was feeling was artificial but certainly meant that what was coming out was being blown up by chemicals in my bloodstream. I cannot explain how precious that interaction was to me. She stayed by my bed until I closed my eyes. I saw the same nurse a few days later and I attempted to thank her, she quickly interrupted my sentence and said gently "we've sorted that and if you need anything else, just ask."

My favourite Nurse was a woman called Sarah. She had a wicked sense of humour and whilst she only worked a few days a week she always had great craic. Her husband had suffered from back problems and had been operated on by Mr Quiet. This gave her a personal understanding to my condition which enhanced her treatment of me tenfold. Sarah would share videos of her at an adult gymnastics class doing human pyramids and floor work. She listened to me on my bad days and was the big advocator of prune juice and its digestive wonders, The thing I like most about Sarah was her ability to take the surroundings of the ward and bounce of it with positive energy. This was not pretend but came from a burning desire to help those around her. Sarah had such a profound effect on me I felt the urge to message her after I left the hospital to try and vocalise my gratitude. Being a bit creepy I found her on the dreaded social media platforms and sent a message of thanks. I opened with a deep apology if it was inappropriate to do this, as I am sure someone somewhere has caught attention in the wrong sense but in my case it was met with the compassion she had practiced every day on the ward. The first thing she replied with was that the feedback form I had filled in (where I had named her and a few others) had received her commendation from the Boss Sister. She then added: "To be honest, when we can have people who we can talk to and have a bit of a laugh with, it makes our job so much nicer and you were certainly one of those people! Always polite and patient, even in extreme pain. A pleasure to care for. I truly hope you continue to improve and make a full recovery for what has been a very difficult time for you, and from this experience you will gain strength not only in body but in mind and spirit!!"

These words filled my soul with happiness. Even after I was out of the hospital Sarah was continuing to support and nurture me. These words are something I hope to use as a mantra when healthy, to use the dark as a starting block running towards the light, rather than somewhere to just to sit and hide. I am so blessed to have met Sarah and every nurse on my ward in the NHS hospital. They are overworked, underpaid and far more vital to the United Kingdom than any Brexit deal. The nurses who work in the NHS are the sparks that keep the whole machine working. Whilst in an NHS hospital, the nurses were all compassionate, human, kind and extraordinary and I would like to personally thank all of them, it is such a shame however that our government does not feel the same and refuses to give them the training, resources and financial support their work truly deserves.

Exits

Three weeks in hospital had dragged by like a maths lesson in year nine. Meals came on trays laden with instant custard and little pots of jelly (strawberry was my favourite), patients came and went and getting a sound night's sleep was as easy as getting a ticket to Glastonbury. Like a Mexican standoff, Smokey and I were the last rangers in the saloon, much to the disappointment of hospital management. My morning started in the usual manner of watching to see a group of people approaching Smokey's bed and they were holding clipboards, which always meant trouble. Curtains drawn and the interrogation began.

Next to Smokey's bed was a window, the very one he has been smoking by on my first night. This window overlooked a portion of rooftop which was secluded and only accessible via Smokey's window. Earlier that morning, a nurse had noticed an empty vodka bottle smack bang in the middle and the clipboard brigade had one suspect in mind. True to form Smokey channelled his inner performer and denied all allegations that were hurled at him. He pleaded that he was innocent and asked to be breathalysed to prove this (which it wouldn't if he had drunk it early enough in the night.) The problem was that all this evidence was circumstantial and although there was no way that bottle had got onto the roof than from the window, no one had seen him throw it out. I assume this was the smoking gun the hospital had been waiting for to finally get Smokey out of his bed. The questioning was not direct and was angled in a manner that was supportive to man with an addiction. "I am concerned about your drinking and would like to offer you some support." Smokey was taken by this gesture, as I presume people normally lead with much more aggressive lines of questioning. He went quiet for a moment holding the room in the palm of his hand and just when we thought we were going to be surprised, he started aggressively defending himself claiming no evidence and that this had become a witch hunt.

I pondered whether they had seen the discarded beer cans in the bathroom or found some other piece of damning information. In theory you could blame any man on this ward for the empty drinking vessels as I always saw them in the bathroom which we all used. I could not figure this one out as I had seen Smokey drunk on the ward most nights, but I cannot believe he would be stupid enough to throw it on the roof where he knew it would be in plain sight. I held enough evidence to stand trial as a key witness but kept my mouth firmly shut as I had seen flashes of a fiery temper in Smokey and I wanted to avoid that at all costs. The integration was over, and they took photographs of the bottle on the roof and announced they would return later with an update. "Can you believe that mate?" Smokey immediately asked me "yes" I thought and "no" I answered aloud. Entering into the well of gossip I had to listen to a man obsessed with a system that was out to get him. From my bed it always looked like he had been treated respectfully even when the odds were stacked against him. What I never figured out was how Smokey had got his this far without being caught. The bins were changed twice a day, so I cannot have been the only witness to the cans. After he finished his anti-establishment lecture he raised up and headed outside for a cigarette whilst I tucked myself for a midmorning nap.

Later that afternoon the verdict was in. Smokey was told he would be moved to another ward which was for people close to being discharged and who required less urgent care. It was interesting that they did not mention the bottle on the roof which was to be removed by a porter later that day. Using the guise of care, they explained that his bed was for someone worse off and hence Smokey was moving on. He did not complain and was given a few hours to pack his things. Another ward was still not the outside world so in my opinion he was still contented. Just before he departed, he wheeled over to my bedside and spoke to me gently. "Just wanted to say mate, thanks for everything. We have been through a lot and you and me and have been here since day one. I'll be sure to come and visit you because I'm only downstairs. I also have some sandwiches which you can have, oh yeah, and these are for you." With this he passed me a pack of wine gums which had the top two missing. "Thank you" I replied and then he shook my hand and smiled at me and that was the cue to exit stage left pursued by an addiction therapist.

I spent more time with Smokey than anyone else in that hospital. He was crass, blunt, an alcoholic and an ex con but he was still a human being. A man that society has forgot, or just let fall through the cracks. I knew he had nothing in material possessions, family support or even a safe place to call home but here he was handing me a packet of confectionary. This gesture sat well in my heart and in that moment, I forgave him for everything he had put me and my ward colleagues through. He had made the stay eventful and you must hand it to him, he was anything but boring. I never saw Smokey after that day but my thoughts often ponder if he will see his estranged children and wife again, or whether he will stay in the system until it all falls down around him.

The next morning after breakfast, it was my turn to be visited by the clipboard gang. As soon as the Boss Sister approached me, I accepted my fate and just complied. The accident and emergency department were swelling and they desperately needed my bed. This was not a forceful move but instead a request if they could get me home it would make a real difference to someone's health. By this time the drugs had made my pain more manageable mainly because I was off my tits dawn until dust. I could not walk but my surgery was four days away and if I could lay in bed here, I could do so at home as there was not much more, they could do for me. I agreed to be discharged on the basis they got me home and into the house and ALL the drugs were given to me so I could survive until the big cut. They had no problem with my request and told me it would take the day to organise and I should expect to go home later that afternoon.

I had been saving a card in my bedside table for this exact day. I scribbled some sentiment and addressed it to the Boss sister. Trying to name and thank everyone who helped me in the ward was impossible, so I generalised but asked she mention it at a staff meeting. Three and a half weeks is a pretty good run for someone in hospital and I can honestly say that the ward will change me for the rest of my life. The people I met, the feelings I felt and the tears I cried are all good stock in enabling me to be a better human being in the future. I packed up my possessions and waited for the hospital transport to come and pick me up. My drug sack was handed over with a short essay on how and when I should take them. My chariot arrived and I was hoisted onto a flat stretcher and strapped in like those who are lifted by a rescue helicopter. They wheeled me out of the ward but all I could see the ceiling blur past my eyes. Thoughts of my mother flooded my mind as when she made the same journey I did, she died the following day. I was not to share the same fate, but I kept thinking if she knew that from her body what was about to happen. Todd had left hospital and may well now have passed on. Matt would be at home with his fiancée planning a wedding he was risking all to get to. Hopefully screaming man's stomach had healed and he was back to form. All the people I had met along the way had lent me insights into existence that was foreign from my young mind. I had witnessed strength, compassion and a man smoking a cigarette inside a ward full of sick men. I had seen it all and had survived it because I was one of the lucky ones if that makes any sense at all...

I arrived at home and was carried on a stretcher up the drive and into the house causing quite the stir with anyone walking by. I was to occupy the spare room as sleeping in my partner's bed was not safe. It felt strange being back at home in comfortable surroundings and a place where you had privacy and no more blue curtains revealing everything to those around you. I was deafened by the quiet that engulfed the room and for a moment I missed the ward. This was interrupted by my partner's mother arriving upstairs with a. cup of tea and a smile. She then helped me make a chart of when I needed to take the drugs, organised into times and dosage. This was then drawn in a grid system making it easy to follow and step by step. I could tell she was worried by the number of drugs I had been given and this was not an overreaction because I had enough stock to begin shooting the *Scarface* Sequel. It is quite staggering how much I had been given to take home and sometimes I would consider what would happen if I swallowed all of them and just closed my eyes, would it be gently into that good night or an explosion of vomit, foaming mouth and a slow and painful end? I must be clear that I was not considering killing myself in these moments, but I would liken it to thinking what would happen if I had ten bottles of wine right now, would I stomach it or just pass out? When you are unwell, you spend a huge amount of time doing nothing and this leads to wandering thoughts to avenues in your imagination you never noticed before. Lewis Carroll called this the rabbit hole and I think there is some truth in it because once you're inside, you have no idea where the end or beginning is. You are tumbling into the abyss, hoping the curiosity that lead you here comes good.

I survived being at home without little incident, but this was because I did not leave my bed. The bathroom was across the hall and with the wall's support I could manoeuvre it quite easily. My NHS nursing team were replaced with my partner's family who cooked for me, brought me drinks and even little bowels of fruit to keep my snacking healthy. I was so lucky to be cared for like that. It made me think of Smokey and where he might be, or if he was with anyone who was keeping him on the straight and narrow.

In my first week of hospital the Physio team had told me that following my discharge this would automatically activate a home visit by the care team. Their job was to come into my home surroundings and asses the surroundings. They were also to offer advice on safety in terms of stairs and potential hazards. I never received such a visit which was disappointing, but I had a secure plan: stay in bed which is to be safe in bed. I think this lapse was due to the haste in which I was discharged and maybe some aspect of that missed something on the system. No matter in my mind as this did no harm. I was deep into a new John Grisham book and at this point I was just happy to be in a peaceful environment.

Enter Hospital 2.0

I was to report to the private hospital by 3pm on the first day of May 2019. I had been given instructions to eat nothing that day and only drink liquids up until 10:30am which was simple as my stomach was violently swelling with butterflies. I was terrified but tried to focus all my energy on the final hurdle, one more leap and I would be on the home straight and across the line. My Father and stepmother had kindly offered to drive me over to the hospital which meant a huge amount to me. The familiar amongst the unknown calms the noise and after all they had done this was another gesture of love as it would include a 250-mile round trip. As if paying for the procedure was not kind enough, their company was worth even more.

For the second time in ten days I entered the shiny hospital without claiming a free mocha which pissed me off. As I clocked the machine by reception, I made a mental note that I would ask for one later, as if that would be my first priority following spinal surgery. The lady at the desk was polite as my father announced, "my son is here to check in for his operation." The receptionists were all dressed in a trendy uniform with a scarf around their necks. Think British Airway's flight attendant for a similar look. I say BA because their first-class cabins would be the best way to describe the room that I would be based in. The room was like a 4* hotel. My bed was in in the middle of a spacious ground floor garden view room. I had a massive flat screen television attracted the wall with a glass bottle of iced water on my side table. Left of the bed were two plush leather armchairs with a coffee table between them. The bathroom had a power shower, toilet and basin with all the shampoos and creams you would expect in a Hilton Hotel. This was very different to the six-man open plan home in my previous hospital, mostly so in decibels. It was so peaceful in this room, a perfect spot to get through my upcoming ordeal. As my father helped me into bed, I thought that it was a shame I was here to be cut open and not for a holiday. The only thing missing from this room was a fluffy dressing gown and bottle of champagne.

Part of my preparation for coming into hospital was to bag all my medication into clearly labelled boxes and sit them in a spacious freezer bag. I also added my handmade drug chart for extra credit with teacher. Private nurse arrived in a bright green outfit and explained that she would be doing the usual observations. "Would you like to have my medication" I added as she wrapped the blood pressure armband around my bicep. "That is fine for now, just leave it on the side." This set off a little alarm bell in my head. I was on a lot of medication, most of which my body was desperately addicted to. Any change to my perfected schedule could have adverse reactions. I looked over at my stepmother and she gave me a glance as if to say "leave it Craig, they are the professionals." I was used to the diligence of the NHS nurses who never missed a trick and to come across a nurse who seemed relaxed and uninterested in me, was a worry. I was not in Kansas anymore, or maybe I was, and the NHS was Oz, but either way this nurse did not grab my trust. She finished all the checks, gave me a series of forms to sign and exited.

Mr Quiet shuffled in next. Dressed in a navy suit and a red tie, he looked the business which was reassuring. My father put his hand confidently forward to which Mr Quiet did not meet but instead awkwardly said "hello" without making any eye contact. "Do you have any questions for me?' was his first sentence he spoke. This took me by surprise as I expected medical formalities or at the very least an update since I had seen him three and a half weeks ago. "No" I answered firmly mirroring his talents for lavish conversation. He then whipped out the consent forms for the operation which I scanned and scribbled on. These basically give legal permission for the operation and if I was to die from an infection or any other possible complication, Mr Quiet would not be legally responsible. I considered what was out of this bracket and it all went wrong, when he would be responsible, after all he is the only one cutting me open? The exchange was closed with the most basic schoolboy explanation of what was going to happen followed by a confident remark that showed he had this in the bag and it would all be sunshine and rainbows soon. I respected Mr Quiet hugely as his simple communication techniques removed the enormity from the room and just kept it simple. I did not need to know the intricate levels of his surgical actions and what was being cut and how. I just needed to know he was up for it and that was enough. For me, being low key kept this relaxed which was a blessing at this moment. He then left my room and tagged in his partner Mr Flash, my anaesthetist (the man who would put me to sleep on the table.)

The gold watch on Flashes' wrist lit up the room like a flare and was a quick reminder of the remuneration of private healthcare. Mr Flash shook everybody in the room's hand and was charming in decorum that would have seen him go well in a sales career. "We will put you to sleep and then once Mr Quiet has finished, we will take you to recovery and wake you up. Once you are stable then you will leave recovery and be brought back here to recover." That all sounded like a summer breeze until he asked me about the medication I was currently on. My father handed him my science homework which had all the information that was required. Mr Flash was silent as he absorbed my lazy handwriting. "Gosh, you are on a heck of a mixture. How long has it been like this?" "My meds have changed as my pain got worse, but the super strong ones have been for a few months now" I replied. "I see" Flash added as he looked puzzled at the list once again.

The reason for his concern was that the medication they would normally use to relieve me when I wake up from surgery was much weaker than what I was taking regularly. By having all these drugs in my body for so long, it meant that I had built up a strong tolerance against them. Being Mick Jagger meant that giving me weaker drugs than what I was taking normally would not kill my pain. Mr Flash was concerned, and it was written all over his face. This would mean that when he brought me round, they would need to use stronger drugs than they normally would for this procedure. I trusted the experts because there was nothing I could have done differently up to this point. The medication had become a fundamental part of my life and whilst they relaxed the pain in my leg, they never got rid of it. "Do you think this will be a challenge (couldn't use problem with Dad in the room)?" I nervously spoke. Shining like the gold wrist accessory he warmly smiled "not at all Craig, just good to be aware of everything." Checking I was ok, Flash then shook everyone's hands again and was off. Elvis had left the building and I was less an hour away to having the muchly anticipated operation.

Private nurse returned with my evening's garments. These included a turquoise gown that opens from the back with white draw strings and a pair of thin white cotton briefs that were so fine you could see through. "Please take all your clothes off and put these on" she requested. Looking at these materials I wondered if they were new, or had been recycled and washed after hugging other people, had anyone died in these? This was a silly thought but much of what goes on in my head is beyond sensical. My stepmother took leave in an attempt to rescue my devastated dignity as my father dressed me for battle. History repeated itself as a dad clothed his son, but we are never too old to accept some help from our beloved family. Dressed ready for my episode of Scrubs I was handed the final piece of the puzzle. Private nurse passed two menus for me to select my dinner and breakfast choices. I chuckled as I opened the laminated cardboard selection that would be better suited in Café Rouge than a hospital. This menu was full of treats and my empty stomach rumbled. Meat, fish, Vegetarian, Salads and sandwiches all smiled at me. I went for the conservative option in a chicken salad sandwich and crisps with a coke.

I had a feeling that after my operation food would not be the main desire so safe was a wise choice. Throwing caution to the wind, I circled Crumpets, jam, Granola and Greek yoghurt and a pot of black coffee for my morning meal. All that was missing was a Bloody Mary or a glass of prosecco. "Worth the seven grand, right?" I joked, as my gag fell flat on the audience. Tough crowd guys, I am about to have spinal surgery here, the least I expected was a sympathy laugh. The nurse interrupted my stand-up routine and notified me they would come and get me soon to go up.

Fate has waved its wand over my family many times to varying emotions. I am not going to write that we have always got on because that would be a lie. Relationships are complicated in your clan and managing these can be a delicate operation. Sat in silence I looked at the man and the woman who were responsible for making this operation possible. Without them I would have been stuck at home, crippled and addicted to powerful drugs for at least three more months whilst I waited for an NHS operation by the same man working here. I was scared, emotional and humbled by the selfless act of these two people in saving my life. I had lost my job, become disabled and if I am being totally frank, contemplated the worth of my existence in my broken body. Reading my mind, my father stood up and walked to my bed side. "We will be right here." The man of thousand words was limited to this. My Stepmother looked over at me with eyes that showed her love in a family that was not blood but had become her own. The room was deafening with noise, but no one was talking. "I love you" left my trembling lips as the door was wrapped with a solemn knock. "They are ready for you" plagued the room and with that I was away for an op.

Recovery

Laying on the meat slab with Kool and the Gang surrounding me, I was certainly the centrepiece. Mr Quiet and Mr Flash were now in green scrubs and gowns with masks and hats on looking very surgical. A female voice asked me to confirm my full name and date of birth, so they were not cutting into the wrong person. I counted five people in the room who were all very busy now doing things which was stressing me out. The activity surrounding me was confusing as you are trying to figure out what it means, or who is doing what? You are aware of what is about to happen and what it involved. I was curious and wanted to know who oversaw the scalpels, who was checking my observations and how they were going to get me on my front as I was wide awake resting on my back? The ceiling was white and clinical. My nose was filled with odd smells and I was terrified. I did not want to do this anymore and the moment controlled me. Reality was here and I was trembling. Those around me must have sensed my trepidation and I bet they all thought how pathetic I was. I hated this and I hated my stupid body for leaving me with a bulge on my discs and all the crap falling from my own personal rain cloud. From the sky came something else which did not smell like crap "here is some oxygen for you, take a deep breath" Mr Flash told me as he held the breathing mask over my mouth and nose. One puff. Two puffs and on the third the ceiling turns blue and like that, my eyes were out for the count and fast asleep.

The next thing that I was aware of was someone speaking my name very softly in an annoying pitch. A ghostly echo penetrated my ears. My eyes were still closed, and my body felt as if it were made up of marshmallow rather than flesh. "Craig, can you hear me? Are you awake Craig?" This voice was sharp to listen to. With each repeated sentence slashing like butcher's knife at the pig's belly. I just wanted to keep sleeping as that was the deepest sleep I had experienced in recent memory. "Let me lie here and sleep" I answered in my mind. For all my resistance the voice would not go away and was getting louder. The marshmallow was turning to a dense solid and suddenly I was aware of something that was very wrong. In the centre of my body was a feeling I can only describe as hell's mouth. A raw, tender, slashing and throbbing pain that forced my first words to be a loud shriek in agony. I was now awake and lying on a bed in recovery having not died in surgery.

Coming around I was very confused. You do not immediately remember how you came to be where you are. The two women speaking my name I had never seen before and all I could see were the siblings of my old friend, the green paper curtains. The pain I was feeling was getting worse and I could not just lay here and accept it because my body was panicking. I decided that the best course of action was to get up and out of bed to have a walk around, stroll it off as going a for walk always helped those people in the films. So I tried to lift my torso from the bed and a hot poker of molten steel exploded in my lower back causing me to flail my arms almost hitting the woman to my left in the face. It was a stunning dodge that would have sat well in UFC. I was now very agitated and still trying to get out of bed, despite the fact there was a five-inch hole in my back being held together by seven metal staples. The women were trying to calm me down and were now holding my arms to stop me lifting my chest up. They managed to rest both hands on my shoulders and pin me down. "How is your pain?" the lady on my left asked me who I think was in charge. "25" I shouted. The NHS has a pain scale of 1-10 which was asked to describe how you are feeling and although putting a value on a feeling is problematic, it was the best they had. The private hospital I was now in worked on a basis of 1-4 instead, which made no sense to me. The lady explained the new scale to me and repeated the question. "25" I answered. This was not a pain, but a demon possessing my body and it was too much to handle. Everything was painful, even breathing. All I wanted was to get up and walk out and all would be fine because if I did that my deluded mind explained the pain would disappear. Following my exaggerated rating of my pain the lady to my left attached a plastic syringe to a line in my hand. She emptied the clear liquid with purpose, and I watched it like a cut bleeding inside you. They were clearly expecting this to calm me, heal me or at least stop me from being such a dick, but unfortunately the latter was in my blood and the first two were unaffected. This process was repeated and with an optimism that would soon be smashed for six. The Fentanyl (a synthetic opiate that in some forms is stronger than Heroin) that was being pumped into my body was doing nothing for my pain and the younger woman was starting to look at her colleague with darkening concern.

Thirty minutes which would have passed longer than the seventh season of Game of Thrones to me, and the team next to me were stumped. They had added some other chemicals into the mix, they had attached a mask to my face with some air, and they were stroking my hair. I was a wreck. Barely able to speak and answering with monosyllabic utterances, I was dominated by the torment in my body and I can vividly remember thinking that my back was broken for good and those small percentages that I had disregarded in Mr Quiet's office were about to define my life. Enter Mr Flash and he swoops in to try and help. He throws a barrage of questions in my direction to which I am unable to answer, but I do remember asking him "can I get up out of bed?" Looking back, I can see that the pain was confusing me and my obsession with walking and leaving the room was a fantastic one. He rubbed my arm and spoke to the two women about further courses of action. They left me for a few moments and returned. More drugs went in and slowly but surely, I began to take stock of my surroundings:

You're in recovery Craig. You have just had your lower back cut into, and you've just woken up from general anaesthetic. The pain inside your body is where they cut through three layers of skin and muscle to get to your spine. These two women are trying to help. You cannot stand up and need to lay still and let these people help. I repeat. Let these people help you. Also apologise for almost hitting her, that's really poor form.

Craig was back in the room, barely. I took the mask off my face as I felt like I was suffocating and was given a little tube with nose holes to replace it. "The oxygen will help" the lady to my right told me. "You gave us quite a scare but you're alright Craig, everything is going to be alright." She held my hand and then it hit me. I did recognise this woman; she was in the room before I went under. I also remember that what Mr Flash had claimed was oxygen was far from O2 and was the magical potion which sent me into a deep abyss. I was filled with a burden of shame, especially as I had nearly smacked one of the staff in the face. I started to apologise profusely and the two women could not have been more sympathetic. "People try and hit us all the time" she joked, and I felt as funny as a man jumping on someone's open casket in a funeral home.

I cannot be the only person who has freaked out post-surgery, but no one had warned me. Mr Flash had correctly predicted what would happen after my operation but had not shared details. The reason my body was in such shock was because the drugs they gave me were not strong enough for the pain. I woke up with the equivalent of no pain killers in my system after having spinal surgery. My tolerance was so high from everything that had I had taken that it took an abnormal amount to make me comfortable. As the pain was slipping away so was reality and it came to be that I was now off my face and as high as a kite. I felt invincible. No leg pain, no surgery pain, no life pain because I was flying across the rainbow on my chariot made of Haribo. Everything was now fine and fixed so we can all head to Soho for a raucous night out.

I was in recovery for ninety minutes and this was much longer than expected. Outside the theatre my father had begun to panic because no one was keeping him informed with useful sentences like "your son has just woken up from surgery and is in so much pain and confusion, he doesn't know where he is and wants to go on a walking tour of the hospital." Having now been on the inside one can understand why relatives get the PG 13 version of events. As he had no news, he tried to slip into recovery when another patient was being wheeled out to try and find me. Whilst this was really stupid idea because recovery is a sterile zone and has strict rules upon entry based on this, I loved that man when I heard of his heroics. He knew something was wrong and nothing was going to stop him helping his son. I think it is much more harrowing on those outside the operating theatre than the patient. You are asleep and unaware of time, where for those waiting for you must watch every second drag by like an ageing tortoise. If you are waiting for that Amazon prime delivery, every stir outside your front door can prick your ears, usually to an unsatisfactory outcome. Waiting for a loved one must be agony. If time moves faster when you are having fun, then standing around whilst someone you love is being cut open must be damn laborious. My operation was supposed to last forty-five minutes, and then a cheeky wakey wakey and I would be back in the room. In total I took nearly four hours which must have been agonising for my family. Aside from the waiting is the concern that must also pollute thoughts. If most of us are honest, we do not understand what the elements of spinal surgery are, even if they are explained. We don't need to. The unknown can be terrifying, and the longer I was in there, the more thoughts of error and complication must grow. Days after my surgery I would learn that my father did everything he could to get an update on my condition from asking everyone from the cleaner to the staffing manager. I think there should be a rule if you are in there longer than the allotted time someone should let the family know, maybe that rule exists but was not in play that afternoon.

I had a lot of apologies to make. Having now been made stable in recovery, I immediately remembered my actions in the previous minutes. I began a long speech of regrets, but the woman who had almost caught a right hook, simply held my hand and said, "you gave us a scare there." I felt so cared for in that moment. After all the confusion, pain and drama, I was back and ready to experience my life pain free. Mr Quiet popped over (love that he comes when all is calm) and tells me "Surgery was a success (recovery wasn't.) We removed the bulges all looks good." He left me and I was ready to be reunited with my family. I thanked the two women who had helped me through hell, and I remember thinking I must come and find them another time to thank them but I never did. The doors opened into the main corridor and my Dad was there. He said nothing but ushered my bed down back to the hotel room like a police convey. I was parked up opposite the plasma television with my stepmother perched on the leather chair. I was feeling high as a kite and unphased by the hole in my back. I took a breath and took a moment to process the events of the last few hours. My father was staring intensely at me with eyes which housed a thousand questions to which my stepmother must have realised and asked gently "how was it?" I started to laugh and told them the course of events.

Up and Out

"Would you like your dinner?" interrupted story telling hour with my family. I was off my face and I think my relations realised this as I must have been slurring my words with detailed images of freaking out in recovery. Dinner arrived on a tray. Chicken salad sandwich on a china plate with cutlery that was really posh. A bottle of coke paired with a glass filled with ice cubes. This meal could have been served on any high street in England. I was not hungry at all (the drugs) but forced myself to eat knowing I had not had anything nourishing for twenty-four hours. I grabbed the coke and drank it quickly as I was very thirsty and had a horrible dry mouth (again the drugs) and polished the bottle swiftly. Then I moved onto my bottle of iced water in a glass bottle with sexual curves on it. I had most of this and still was not satisfied. Seeing that I was clearly distracted, my family took this as their exit. They both shared sentiments of love and departed for their hundred-mile journey home. It made a difference having a familiar face to see when out of surgery, and for anyone that has the same dire experience I would advise have someone to support you if you can. Human connection is as powerful as some painkillers and I am privileged to have people around me.

Now alone I grabbed the water bottle and as the last drop entered my mouth a sudden dilemma hit me: how the hell was I going to empty my bladder if I could not yet get out of bed? Luckily for me, hospitals are well equipped. I pressed my buzzer and the nurse appeared and following my request and returned with what can only be described as a cardboard French horn. The vessel I was to fill was a bowl that is completely covered apart from an angled tube which is where you place one's member inside to relieve yourself. The thing that worried me was that the cardboard looks like it isn't waterproof, and I could imagine it filling up and then becoming soggy and falling apart like an American shopping bag in the rain. The fear of being drenched in my own urine forced me to ask the nurse how it worked? She explained delicately and asked if I needed any help? No, I bloody did not, what was she going to do? Thumb my phallus into the urinal musical instrument, I think not. So true to form, I insisted on doing it myself and in so was doomed from the start. The nurse left and I bet she was full of beans knowing that my stubborn resistance to help would leave me out in the rain. Looking at the container I figured out the best technique, I would just roll onto my side, and away we go. I tried that a few times and my body was having none of it, so I had to decipher the secret of the box. If I angled it downwards I could finish so I tried this and immediately missed the target completely leaving urine on my duvet (in private hospital they give you duvets instead of sheets like in the NHS, silly really as they are much harder to clean and this one has piss all over it.) I tried again and landed a bullseye, and all was going well until I found that I was filling it near to the brim and I was far from complete. Any man will tell you that pausing the flow of urine mid flow is very painful and this was no different. Stopping felt like a dagger going into my lower abdomen but I held it as I placed the full jug on my table and buzzed the nurse again. She removed the evidence and gave me a fresh one which was almost filled up also. Having emptied myself I felt much better and made a mental note to chill out on the fluids, especially as a I had a saline drip in my arm, so I was not going to die of dehydration anytime soon.

The bed-based bathroom activities had left me tired but not sleepy. Assuming the fault of the powerful chemicals flowing around my body, I was wired wide awake. A little later on my partner and her mother popped in baring gifts of a chocolate nature. It was great to see them, and I suppose the same could be said for them as a physical visit confirmed I had not died in surgery. We had a short conversation as I imagine I looked worse than I felt. This engagement filled my heart with happiness once more and the trauma of recovery was slipping into darkness. They told me they would come and collect me sometime tomorrow when I was cleared to go home and left me to it. I sat in the room munching on my dinky deckers' flicking through the television channels in in front of me. I came across a Channel Four Documentary where misbehaving teenagers were sent to an American jail and live there as mock prisoners. This was highly amusing, especially one boy who was essentially a spoilt little shit who had been spoilt by his parents and started crying as soon as he arrived in detainment. Others were from harder backgrounds, but I scoffed as the older generations do at the ones behind them thinking 'they don't know how good they have it.' I actually believe there is much truth in my case, because we were the last generation to grow up without smart phones and Facebook, both of which came in when I was 17. Mind you, we did have Zelda, Ocarina of time, and the Water Temple remains one of the hardest things I've ever had to complete.

Throughout the evening nurses and the night doctor had popped in to check my observations and condition. These were the normal checks that made sure everything was on track. I am told that they monitor you closely after surgery because if anything has gone wrong it does so very quickly, so often is better. Compared to the NHS hospital they had much more staff. The doctors were available within minutes and not hours all from a press of a buzzer. This is obviously about funding and I imagine if the NHS had half of what the private sector makes fundamental differences could be made. I have to be honest, I felt guilty many times when in that hospital. I was in a very small bracket of the national population that could afford private healthcare and for the rest, it was wait, and most likely, wait in pain. I tried to remind myself as much as possible of this reality having so recently been in the other camp. I am not sure how much longer the NHS can survive given all the strains on it, but that is not a discussion for now. I just wanted to share that all the attention and lavish care made me very humbled.

After my scathing review of the youth of today was over it was time for Denzel Washington and Dakota Fanning to fill my screen with *Man on Fire*. Quite a gritty film about a girl who gets kidnapped and the revenge story following. I lasted about an hour (which was only about 34 minutes of the film due to adverts) and crashed out. My body must have been exhausted after all it had endured and I drifted off into oblivion. When I woke up, I was suddenly aware of my surroundings with a jagged edge around them. The party was over, and the pain was back, the wound in my spine was on fire again. Panicking I pressed the buzzer and the morning nurse arrived helping me to roll over and inspect the dressing. It was covered in blood (which was normal) and needed changing. I enquired about some pain medication as my button-based morphine machine was now empty and in urgent requirement of refilling. Morning nurse said that my regular nurse would be in before the end of her shift to sort my medication and left to get fresh bandages. Alone and in pain, my breathing quickened, and my eyes filled with tears. It would seem all the drugs from yesterday were gone and my body was waking up to the reality of being at Toby Carvery. I pressed the buzzer, and no one came, the minutes that passed seemed like hours as I trembled in agony and fear. It is in this moment that it does not matter if you are on the NHS or Private, no plush duvet or ensuite is going to cure post-surgical pain, that is the same in either places. The lavish touches don't really make a difference, the medication that kills the pain does. That medication is available in either healthcare systems in the UK and the speedy attention that I enjoyed the night before was now vacant. I submitted to my body and lay there taking it the best I could attempting to distant my mind from my body as a distraction.

Fifteen minutes later, bandage nurse arrived and swapped the dirty for the clean. "Please can I have some pain relief" I begged, "She will be along shortly" she replied. I was beginning to get angry which would only be increased about what followed. Cue the nurse with my pain relief and regular medications. Claiming she has got my dosages from my drug sheet I provided the hospital she handed me the usual paper cup with the tablets inside. As always, my eyes scanned what I was about to swallow when a purple dart hit my retina. In amongst all the white pills was a purple one, which I knew to be Amitriptyline. Side effects include of this nerve pain killer are putting me in coma like sleep for hours, which is why I take it just before I go to sleep in the evening. It was currently seven forty-five in the morning. If I had swallowed the drug, I would have been dead to the world for around five to seven hours. I pointed this out to the nurse who simply remarked "sorry about that, let me double check it shouldn't be in there.' "Please can you check all of the drugs and what should be in there?" I added. The mass mixture of medication I was on needed attention to detail, and this was lacking severely here. I no longer trusted this nurse, so I made her empty the tablets onto the table and we went through what was what compared to my detailed notes. She had only made one error but that was enough. I took the remaining drugs and sulked as I waited on their effects.

I had been in the NHS hospital three and a half weeks and been tended by dozens of nurses. To my knowledge they had not made one error, yet less than twenty-four hours and one nurse could not correctly read a sheet of paper of match that to the medication. I am surely being dramatic, but I was far from impressed. Before coming the private hospital had insisted on a detailed sheet of my drugs so they could be administered correctly. From the moment I met this nurse she had seem relaxed and uninterested in my dosage information and this had nearly cost her a serious plunder. OK, all that would have happened is that I would have been to sleep for a few hours, but this was the morning after surgery. Mr Quiet, the anaesthetist and my physio all had important inspections to do which needed me awake. I was furious and felt unsafe. I laid there with my blood on fire at the nurse's mistake which I put down to lack of concentration. This hospital had plenty of staff, resources and time, none of which was available to the NHS nurses and yet here they were making errors despite their obvious advantages. I am possibly being unfair, as I do not know the mind set of that nurse, but it is not the patient's job to check their drugs, because we are not sound of mind, we have been cut open, remember? I mentioned this to another member of staff a little later and I did not see that nurse again. I also noted this entire incident down in my online feedback form from the private hospital in an attempt to avoid a repeat near calamity.

My morning after surgery had been far from peaceful and this run of luck was to continue when a man in a white polo neck t-shirt appeared and asked me "shall we get you up Craig?" This was going to good. "Sure" I replied. Mr Physio was a beaming man, by this I mean that he had a smile which could fill a room up. His demeanour was kind and he is the type of man you want to be friends with. After the start of my man crush was igniting Mr Physio explained we would stand me up and walk out the door and back to my bed. We were going to use crutches, but this was the first time in testing whether the operation had worked. If I could put weight on my left foot and the pain was calmed and the nerve free of agitation then we were a go, if it was not possible, Houston we have a problem. As I prepped myself for the effort ahead, I was terrified and overcome with self-doubt. Mr Physio sensed this and put me at ease "we don't have to do anything you don't want to but we need to see if Mr Quiet's work has helped." I was eased up to the edge of the bed and I dangled my feet over the precipices. Away I went and I was flooded with a wave of nothing. My leg did not hurt. My back was alight, but I did not care one bit, my leg was pain free and it felt amazing. I was shown how to take gentle steps with the crutches taking the majority of my weight to ease my back pain. My leg was weak and stiff, but it worked and I was back. Plant the crutch, land the second and repeat this with the feet and I was away. After eleven months of a leg swelling with pain I was finally on my way to a real recovery. I must have been walking like someone with a rod or other implement in their behind, but I owned my strut and was mobile once more.

I got back to bed and was dripping in sweat. My hospital gown now wet like the walls after a hot shower. You would assume that one would be ready to celebrate the news of good health loudly and with everyone who would listen. For me, it was the opposite. I sat in bed (painkillers now working) and bathed in the silence. All the noise of hospital wards, cramped GP surgeries, concerned friends or family and the defiant deafening din of sharp pain that manifested in my limbs were all muted. I was at peace for the first time in a year and I sat there planning my new life without any noise around me. That moment was true bliss.

Home Alone

It is amazing how quickly you forget how bad things once were. When you are in severe pain and discomfort you swear to yourself over and over to hold these memories in your body so when they are gone, they can remind you of where you have been and how far you have come. The truth is when good health arrives it is impossible to really immerse yourself in that darkness once more, which is a good thing. I think it is important to use shadows of hardship to fuel one forward but not to hold us back. It is important to take what life throws at you and run with it, or in my case limp around your house whilst your surgical wound heals.

I got home from private hospital without any incidents. The surgery had certainly worked because two days later I was walking without crutches around the house. I was getting up the stairs, I was sitting in a chair and playing loads of FIFA 19. This part of the healing process is not as simple as it might seem. The nerve compression (my Sciatica) had been healed, the compressed nerve released and the leg whilst weak, was pain free. The surgical wound was tender and still had seven metal clips pulling the hole closed that Mr Quiet cut. Alongside this, I was still on a huge number of drugs. The dilemma I found myself in was that the medication I had taken was addictive, very addictive. My body would have now been in a state of thinking to itself 'I need these drugs to function normally' and this is a very bad place to be in. You cannot just stop the drugs because then the body thinks part of its regular routine is out of sync and it makes you sick. This is called withdrawal and is usually associated with people who take heroin or crystal meth and have no teeth. I was not this glamorous but instead realised I needed advice on how to solve this puzzle. I had an appointment with Mr Quiet ten days after my surgery to remove my staples, so I banked it, kept up the drug schedule and made a note to ask the expert for his advice.

After being in two hospitals recuperating at home was a change. The surroundings calmed me and although you fill the days with Xbox and Netflix, you do it on a regular bed and without medical staff and patients around you. The aspect that I found most difficult to handle was the solace of it all, you have company outside working hours, but in the day on your lonesome one's thoughts can drift. One of the things I struggled with was opening myself back up to social connections. I did this in a rather flamboyant fashion and posted a blog on Facebook that I had written through my experiences. This was an honest non-filtered testimony of the highs and lows. In truth I do not remember writing half of it but once I clicked post, an explosion of communication bombarded me, which in my room, looking at my phone, was very overwhelming. I don't know what I expected posting on social media, but so many people from all areas of my past spoke up. They were touched by my honesty and my strife and wished me well and offered invitations of meeting up when I was healthy. It was kind of people to say such lovely things, but I felt like I was drowning in my room all alone. It was like throwing a ball against the wall and having a hundred bounce back at you.

The one sentence that was in almost every message was:

"I am so sorry for what you have been through."

Being a paid-up member of the dead parent club, I have heard this sentence many times. It is the go-to selection of words when we hear something bad, but what does it actually mean? Apologising is something we speak when we have done something wrong and have some sort of responsibility in the action. I am in a packed pub and whilst holding three beers in the triangle grip and someone turns quickly and knocks the glasses causing beer to spill on them and me. As I am holding the beer, I immediately offer "I am so sorry." Judging on the best kind of people it's a "no, no it's my fault, I wasn't looking where I was going." If they are less favourable you could find yourself offering to buy them a drink as an apology such is the world of pub politics. Saying sorry for me being ill suggests the apologiser was holding the beer, or even charged into me when in truth they are not in the pub at all, they are the other side of the city. I am reading too much into it, but the people who touched my loneliness the most were the simple messages of just asking 'how are you getting on?" So often when bad things happen, we skate around the topic because we cannot handle it. I will never forget at my mum's funeral when after the service my father, sister and I stood huddled together whilst a long line of people passed us and wished us well. The majority of people apologised for our loss, and eight-year-old Craig was confused by this, were they apologising because they had something to do with it? The only person that owed me an apology was Cancer and that was never going to happen. Don't get me wrong, people saying something is better than nothing at all, it is just a choice of words that if you unpack it seems not to fit.

One of my best friend's tragically lost her father long before his time was due. It was awful and naturally had a monumental effect on her life. Having been in her exact position I offered simple advice in two things. The first was just to let her know I was there when she was ready. The second was passing on advice that was gifted to me as a teenager that transformed my perspective of losing a parent "You'll never get over it. You just learn to live with it." This profound statement offered me a pure insight into grief. So many discourses offer us to get over and complete the Nintendo game of death which is farcical. When you lose your parent, it is like a portion of your soul being slashed out of your being. They created you and you carry their legacy. As time moved on, my friend and I would talk about our late parents and agree that they are somewhere watching over us. I admit that I often talk to my mother aloud, the most recent of which was just before my surgery. I am not a religious person but believing in some sort of mystical force that enables my mum to hear me when I talk to her, keeps me sane.

Alongside my social anxiety another feeling that started to wash over me when I was recovering was that of depression. This was unexpected as I presumed the worse was over but being alone in the day and wasting time on screens and lounging around affected me. I had no job waiting for me when I was healed. The Insurance company I worked for in their HR department had hired me on a three-month fixed term contract with the plan of training me up to take over from my manager's duties when she left for maternity. When I fell sick, this screwed this plan up royally, so I imagine I caused them some hassle. I hate the recruitment game and the thought of starting from scratch loomed over me. I had lost all my confidence and had been bed bound and medicated for a long time and would often fanaticise about what normal life would be like? How would I fare on a packed train or would I be able to be on my feet for eight hours a day? All these worries and a million more swamped as a demonic cloud formed over my sky. As I was on my own, I did not talk to anyone, I just bottled it up which is honestly the worst thing you can do. This all exploded as these things always do when something irrelevant happened and I burst into tears in front of my girlfriend. Breaking down I revealed how I had been struggling and just opened my soul. She listened and promised to support me no matter what. These words gave me strength to keep on going and also confirming that I was not alone because all I needed to do was ask for help.

Talking to my girlfriend made me feel bad for judging those people's messages from my post. The fact that people were writing any words was a blessing and to over think it like I did was not fair. Not everyone understands the gravity of what you are dealing with and why would they? Contact is better than no contact, so if anyone you know is going through hell drop them a line and I promise one day they will appreciate (it might not be straight away though.) A problem shared is a problem halved (copyright my Dad) because it forces sunlight through those gloomy clouds.

The final aspect of my life at home recovering is what the drugs were doing to my state of mind. A couple of the tablets can cause depression and although you read this on the box or are told it, you often forget. When you are alone you drift into yourself, starting a dialogue with only one voice playing many parts. The drugs help this like pouring petrol onto an open flame. It is impossible for me to measure how much was me and how much the chemicals, but it is something that is majorly understated. In both hospitals only one healthcare professional informed me that side effects could include depression and that was when I told a nurse "I don't want to be here anymore." If you know it is going to happen, you can prepare yourself for it and do things that keep you uplifted. For example, if you are feeling low then reading a phycological crime thriller is probably not the best idea. My advice for anyone who goes through something similar is do things you love. For me, I wrote my blog, binged Netflix and chatted rubbish to those around me. This stopped me from going into myself where there is nothing but echoes to answer your thoughts. You have to give your body time to recover from the mental and physical trauma of surgery and pain. This will not happen overnight and for me once I fully accepted this fact the days got easier. Speak up, rest and be thankful: The worst just might be over but in my case, shit was about to hit the fan.

Dopesick

Ten days after my surgery and I was back in the private hospital in Mr Quiet's office. I was in a good mood because I had arrived with twenty minutes to spare so I had time to polish off a complimentary mocha. The sweet finish of chocolate and the bitter bite of coffee fizzled on my lips as I sat in front of the man who had cut me open and looked my spine in the eye. After the pleasantries he asked me to stand up and place my hands on the bed in the corner of the room and lift my shirt. He admired his craft with a remark of "healed nicely hasn't it?" I affirmed his comment and he then told me "we need to take those staples out" and before I had a chance to brace myself, Mr Quiet went to work quickly pulling the staples out with plyers. It felt like seven sharp stabs into my lower back and after he was finished he invited me to sit back down at his desk.

Sat with a bonfire of discomfort alight in my wound I had one urgent question on my mind. "What is the strategy for me to come off the drugs?" Mr Quiet looked at me and replied "you need to speak with to your GP about that. I have been doing a lot reading recently and the case of drug addiction in these situations is very serious. There are many alternative routes out there which I am looking into." This really pissed me off for two reasons. The way he deflected the responsibility of helping me with my drug addiction made me feel as if he didn't care or couldn't be bothered to get involved with the less interesting side of healthcare. Secondly, where were all these non-drug options when I was agony and swallowing skittles by the bag? I bit my tongue and just let it wash over me. He was a surgeon and I imagine this was a lesser problem, so I left with fourteen small holes in my back and went on my way.

The minute I got home I called my GP surgery and asked "please can I book appointment to see my doctor? and waited with optimism. "There are no appointments today left." That made sense, as it was halfway through the day. The receptionist then asked me "Is it an emergency?" This fell over me for a moment. Say yes and you're in, say no and you have no appointment. Was my addiction to an emergency and was my life in danger? "No, it's not an emergency." I could have lied but somewhere there is another Craig who has just collapsed at a train station who needs to see a doctor. So, I went home and started to google how I could go about getting myself free from the choker of drug addiction.

I called the next day at the precise hour the surgery opened and was greeted by an automated message: "You are number 17 in the queue." If I had been my father, I may have hung up there and then (very short fuse) but I endeavoured and after thirteen minutes I got through. This time I phrased my dilemma slightly differently "I have recently had spinal surgery and need to talk to a doctor about post-operative care" and like a magic key, the lock opened. There were no appointments (naturally) but I was put on the triage list. This is where the doctor calls you sometime in the day and assess if you need to be seen. They have the control over the secret appointments that you can't book, so it is very important to have a good chin wag with the doctor caller. My chance came at half past three in the afternoon where a tired voice asked me "how can I help you?" I explained in detail my recent events in a short sharp version. The voice responded by questioning me on my pain and movement. I answered honestly as I figure there is no point to embellish. The response was not what I wanted "given you're pain I think if you continue on what you are taking, and we can review it in a week. I will send your prescription down to your elected pharmacy electronically and it will be available within the hour." Despite my resistance this was the end, and he said to book an appointment for a week's time to come in and discuss it in further. Heeding this advice, I called the reception back and repeated the doctor's words "we don't have any appointments available next week" the young lady replied. I was fed up and thanked her and hung up. I was not getting any closer to a drug free lifestyle so went to pick up my pharmacy sack of drugs muttering complaints in my thoughts.

It is not the GP's fault, but they are hugely overworked. In my experience if they can give you a quick and simple fix, they will. The quickest answer to my query was to keep me medicated and safe from danger. I was on way too much just from Mr Flash's remarks and all the fun I had in recovery. My level of pain was nothing compared to pre surgery so being on the same dosage seemed insane. Thinking that I was a big money baller with a PHD in healthcare I decided to figure it out myself. The main thing I needed to get off was oxycodone, which I was taking slow release morning and night and then top ups every two hours (or when I needed it.) My actions were meant with good intentions but what nobody tells you is how horrendous withdrawal is. Aaron Paul in *Breaking Bad* was quite accurate, it consumes you entirely. The best way to explain it is imagining for a moment you are starving. You have been at work all day and you skipped lunch because you had back to back meetings, and it is now early evening. On the way home you pass your favourite fast food restaurant (we all have one, I love pizza and usually pick a chain based on their deals) and they are offering a crazy offer on the dish that sets your heart alight. Your stomach is grumbling, you're exhausted, and you feel as if you need that food, that meal will complete you but you know that last night's spag bowl is in the fridge, so you wander on by. That feeling outside of the restaurant, is withdrawal, because your body, mind and soul yearns to be satisfied. You feel like a jigsaw which is missing the final piece, you feel incomplete. When you don't give your body what it wants it is going to make a lot of noise. These fun symptoms include blinding headaches, anxiety, itchy skin, shakes, sweating, vomiting and diarrhoea. It makes you utterly miserable, but you have to give it time. The temptation to just pop a cheeky pill is so prominent that it is all you think about. Morning and night, I dreamt about drugs with my brain promising everything would be alright if only you just took another. "Give in Craig" was on repeat like a song you hate married with a physical onslaught of sickness. I was bed bound and as useful as a chocolate teapot but I stuck to my guns and managed to wine myself off the chemicals, I was ten days clean and went back to the GP for a check-up because my symptoms were lingering a little longer than normal. Sleeping soundly had become a massive problem, to the point I was becoming an early morning FIFA expert. I also had a tight chest with shortness of breath which is probably because I had done zero exercise in several months, that and I was recovering from the mental and physical trauma of the previous week's experiences.

New doctor with new rules. My withdrawal symptoms were not quite what was normal, whatever that is. Four weeks post-surgery, the wound is healing nicely, and I am doing physio exercises daily to strengthen the lower back. Having spoken to the phone doctor they had ushered me to an appointment. Doctor Interested asked me describe at length my issues and agreed that my tight chest pain was peculiar given the length of time I had been drug free. She listened to my heart and made me do some deep breathing tasks (which made me feel very lightheaded) and finished by checking my neck and down my throat. "You may have a blood clot in one of your lungs, I am going to get you an ECG (electrocardiogram) and a blood test to check. The nurse will see you shortly and I'll call you later with the results." Standing up I felt like I had been here before, as my mind drifted back to the waiting room where nightmares were common and the entrance to hell boiled and brewed. When you are told medical words you freak out, it is a human trait. We fear the unknown, and a lung clot sounds bad, you cannot sugar coat it. Sat there waiting for the nurses beckoning I pondered telling my family that there was more bad news. We had all been through so much, and I had captained the drama. If you had given me this scenario a few months earlier I would be much more out of control but after an initial worry, I brushed it off and thought "couldn't be worse that spinal surgery, could it?"

The nurse that was doing my checks was annoyingly chatty. "Gosh you've been through so much for a young man. What an ordeal it must have been. It must have been so tough. The thing you need to be sure of is looking after that back of yours. Have they gone through any exercises with you?" The one-way dialogue continued as she placed stickers on my chest and back. Some bleeps and the machine printed out a graph on a long strip of paper. Needle in the arm and blood drawn and I was finished for the day. I called my dad on the walk home and brought him up to date. Calling home with persistent bad news must have been wrecking their feelings and I longed to share good news with them both. On the positive my back was healing nicely, and the leg was pain free but the tight chest and insomnia was worrying me. I would not share this with anyone, but I was becoming increasingly aware that something in my body was not right and my gut screamed it had nothing to do with drugs or the spinal surgery. Much later that afternoon Doctor Interested called and explained everything was clear but added "if you are concerned in the future then do call 111 and an ambulance can come and check you out if needed." She prescribed some muscle relaxants which would help me sleep (they didn't) and wished me well.

The experts are the wise ones because of education and experience and healthcare professionals are no different. We trust them based on this logic and my inner voice reminded me of this as I continued to feel crap in the days following my appointment. The pills did nothing for my sleeping, so I spent days drifting like an aimless shadow through rooms of darkness, barely visible and vacant in thought. I could not put my finger on it, but I felt peculiar. Sweating was becoming part of my hourly routine and I lost all sense of emotions. All of this going on inside of me was hidden for fear of complaining too much. For so long I had been the problem child to my girlfriend, her family and everyone around me because it felt like I was drowning. My body had something wrong, but no tests would be able to solve it and you simply start to question your sanity. "Is all this made up because I love being the sick and weak man and all the attention that comes with it?" echoed around my head, was I losing my grip on reality because everything had finally tipped me over the edge? This all came to a climax on the Saturday after seeing Doctor Interested when after trying to sleep for a few hours my chest was tight, my heart racing and I was very cold all over. I rolled over and looked at my phone, it was three in the morning, so I acted on previous advice and dialled 111.

The call did not last long, and after a series of questions and answers they confirmed an ambulance was being dispatched to come and check me out. I woke up my girlfriend and let her know of our late-night visitors. Upon explaining tears appeared on my face under the shame of seeking more medical attention. I felt as if I was playing up to something and acting out. "Am I making all this up?" I asked her, to which she replied with calming sentences of affections. This made me think of when I was a child at school and would see a friend with a broken leg in a cast and think "that would be cool." I don't know why the medical treatment process was something I yearned for, but maybe in some part of my subconscious I was manifesting these bizarre symptoms to satisfy a seven-year old's passion to be trendy. My mind was split and dislodged, so when the ambulance men arrived (within eleven minutes) and confirmed my heart was racing (through a mobile ECG) and my temperature was slightly raised I felt a little better for making a scene. Given the surgery being so recent and fears of links to that healing process, they suggested I went back to hospital for further examination. This was not the news I wanted to hear but the two paramedics insisted and who am I to turn down such a warm reception?

I would travel to the hospital in the back of the ambulance and whilst we drove, the paramedic shared he had suffered with sciatica twice. He instantly emphasised with my situation and the battle with drug addiction and withdrawal. "I stopped taking morphine the day after my operation because I had been on it for eight months and it was the worse decision I ever made" he revealed to me. "How long did it take for the body to repair back to zero?" I asked keenly to which he replied, "months mate." This did not fill me with confidence as I was only weeks into my recovery. We swapped stories of suicidal dreams and not being able to walk which made me relaxed talking to someone who gets the whole picture. After a short drive we arrived at the hospital and I went in via the VIP entrance (ambulance skips the waiting room) and was placed on a bed in my second home. The paramedic who had been so honest with me wished me well and offered a gift of "keep at it mate, you'll be alright." That encounter helped calm my current mental crisis of one's sanity and after he left, and I was on my bed and pondered how many people this condition had burdened and how I could talk to them? Maybe a Sciatica helpline App could be my business venture when getting healthy making me the Zuckerberg of agony aunts for back pain.

Two hours later and the doctor on duty came to see me. They had done a chest X-ray which was clear, and he quizzed me on my current situation in a sugary American accent. He stated that my temperature had come down (probably down to the paracetamol, when you're hot it's good to drop.) His closing remarks linked this all to the drug withdrawal and prescribed me some withdrawal medication and to be fair to my smooth American operator, it made me fill much better. I checked out at eight AM on Sunday morning heading home with a new wave of optimism that the withdrawal would be a five-day test rather than a 20/20 cricket match, and I needed to grin and bear it. This realisation would not last long as the next week would smash all the theories out of the window and descend me into hell's inferno once more. Upon reaching home, I collapsed into a much-needed sleep unaware of the hurricane on my horizon.

Enter Hospital 3.0

Murky Monday arrived with silent applause. Waking up and my body was up to something I just could not put my finger on. Having been given the all clear by the hospital I thought twice before dialling my GP surgery and asking for an emergency appointment but stuck with my gut. My body was the king of surprises and maybe this party trick was a red herring, but my mind concentrated on the withdrawal sickness bubbling in my soul. My local surgery is a short walk and as I ambled over, I took stock of my two feet that can move in unison to propel me forward. This simple task had escaped me in the depths of Sciatica and although I felt like crap, I gave a blessing for my good fortune. This tiny air bubble of positive energy was overcome by my sickness because after everything I had been through, was I really going to have something else wrong with me? My life was becoming a Noel Coward play replacing country homes with hospitals and an upper-class family with what seemed like the entire countries healthcare system. "Your temperature and blood pressure are normal, and I can only attribute your sickness to your body still struggling with withdrawal" explained the bemused GP. He then set about prescribing me a nerve pain killer in the same dose that I was on in hospital. "I don't have any nerve pain, why would I take these?" I asked in dismay, "Your body could be reacting to the addiction to Pregabalin, so by putting you back on it, this might help with your symptoms" Doctor bemused told me. Fix withdrawal from drugs by taking more drugs that you were in withdrawal from in the first place in a hope it all fixes itself. On a good day I would I have questioned this insane logic but instead answered "what about my sleeping problems?" Bemused scribbled something down and I was away to the pharmacy. I picked up my sleeping pills and nerve drugs and made my way home. The walk back was slow as my head felt as if a beachball was being inflated up and down whilst smashing against my skull. I was dripping in sweat and could not really focus. Arriving home I swallowed the pregabalin (nerve drugs) and noticed on the box it read "this medication may make you sleepy" which was true because at around midday I sat down to play Xbox and was dead to the world in under ten minutes.

Sleeping beauty was roused from bed by a loud wrapping on the front door at around three in the afternoon. Lifting myself from the duvet I suddenly realised the room was spinning. I answered the door to a delivery man and then entered the bathroom to inspect my face. My eyes were bloodshot, I was freezing cold and my headache was out of control. Feeling lightheaded and sick, I felt out of control of my body and immediately called my GP surgery stating that my symptoms were much worse and that I was freaking the hell out. Whether it was the panic in my voice or a slow Monday, but I was given the last appointment of the day with Doctor Bemused who had seen me earlier. That gave me three hours to figure what on earth was going on? I immediately put on a jumper and a coat and lay on the kitchen floor sipping water. I could not control my body trembling and I fumbled with my phone to call my girlfriend. Within sentences I broke down in an explosion of tears and fears to which she confirmed she would leave work and come home immediately to my rescue. I have not given enough praise to my girlfriend in these pages, but this is one in dozens of examples of her selfless love. Every time I have really needed her, she has been there, and I am incredibly lucky to have someone like that at my side. Like a scene from *Fear Unloading in Las Vegas* the familiarities of the kitchen became obscure and bizarre. Pain and confusion swirled around my body and mind as I lay there waiting on help's arrival.

Within the hour my partner arrived finding me on the kitchen floor shaking and in a heck of state. Upon early conversation I muttered a phrase that had once before left my lips "I don't want to be here anymore." This sentence was more me expressing my total loss of faith in that moment. I had no energy left in my failing body to fight anymore and in that beat of my life, I honestly wished I was not alive. It is terrifying to look back on but when you are sick, in pain and on the end of a long journey there has to be a breaking point, and this was mine. Like Frodo and his fellowship, the burden was not just mine to carry and my other half got me up and just hugged me tight and promised "everything will be alright" and whilst I heard the words, I did not believe her.

Layered up like an Eskimo we went to the GP surgery for the second time in a day and waited for my appointment. Sitting on the chair was impossible in my state of health, so I just set myself up by lying flat on the ground and waited for my name to be called. There were a few people in the room who I am sure were curious why a man was lying face down on the floor but all too polite to comment.

Every single appointment I have had in this building has had an average of running twenty minutes late and this was no different with me being the last of the day, half an hour after my allotted time. "Hello Craig, I can see things have not improved since this morning" was my greeting from Doctor Bemused to which I just nodded my head. I wanted to ask him why he had given me that drug or what was wrong with me but just stared at the GP with a hazed glare. Sensing I was not going to be the chatty type, my girlfriend suggested he take my temperature as my forehead was on fire and I felt as cold as a cornetto. The sensor in my ear revealed I had a temperature of 40.5 which to put in context, my normal and healthy temperature would be 36.5. This showed I had a fever which meant my body was fighting like mad, but the look on the doctor's face when he read my score was anything but bemused. "You need to go to the hospital and you need to go right now" he instructed urgently as he again did my temperature to reveal the same figures. "I know this is the last thing you want to hear Craig but I think something is very wrong and you need to be checked out" the doctor added. Relieved that my sickness was not totally whimsical we left the surgery and headed back to where I had been so many times in the last few months. The last thing Doctor Bemused had gifted me was a letter explaining his findings which I presented at the check in desk to a woman in crimson who taking one look at me figured things were not too well. The hospital screen glared a two-hour waiting time which I hoped would not be the case. It was strange sitting here because for the first time I had no wish or care about what was wrong with me because feelings of disappearing sung a song on repeat.

Feeling down and out and I embraced my fever lifestyle shivering away. A mixture of what had come before mixed with a continual run of bad luck had left me negative, hopeless and void of emotion. Neither happy nor sad, the familiar surroundings may as well fallen in on me because my heart could not have cared less.

Honestly couldn't tell you how quickly I was called in (for once) but they did call me. The nurses did the normal checks which confirmed my GP's discovery was correct. They took my blood and a doctor came in to have a chat. "It looks like you have an infection so we are going to give an IV of antibiotics whilst we wait for the bloods which will tell us a little more." he explained as the nurse attached a couple of bags of clear liquid to enter my me via the veins in my left arm. Having needles stabbed into me had become quite normal which was curious as it had once made me squirm. Lying there I fully expected to be packed up and out within a few hours as I had been a few days earlier. Imagining the drugs would work their magic I longed to just climb into bed and shut out this all hating world. The doctor returned a few hours later with an update. "Your inflammation marker is off the scale, this probably means you have a very nasty infection which explains the sickness, headache and temperature. Given you have had surgery recently in your spine, I have contacted the Orthopaedic team to come and speak to you, but we will be admitting you this evening to monitor your condition." They knew what the problem was and nothing he said to me alarmed me in anyway. The Doctor left and I told my girlfriend it was OK to leave me. No doubt they would move me to the ward soon and she had work early doors, so we hugged, and she wished me well. Thirty minutes after her departure another woman came in to speak to me. She introduced herself as a doctor from Hungary who was doing a period of work over here in England, which I took as a sabbatical. This woman had an air of serenity around her and for the first time in that day I was about to be caught off guard. "Craig, I am here to talk to you about your infection. We have been discussing it and there is a possibility the it is from the operation on your spine. It could be an abscess, but we won't know until we have an MRI." This Doctor was not part of the Orthopaedic team and I did not understand why she was here, where was my usual doctor? "You need to prepare yourself" she added and looked at me with eyes that caught my soul and locked its attention in. "What do you mean prepare, prepare for me what?" I asked quietly. "Prepare yourself because this could be quite serious." This left me dumbstruck as I had no idea if this was subtext for something else, whether they knew what was wrong me and would not reveal it, or if prepare yourself meant that my life was now in danger? My mind was suddenly alert with questions darting across a head rife with pain. Wanting to know the answer to the most important question, "am I going to die?" left my mouth. "We won't know more until we have the full test results, but I want to you to know that we are here to support you through this." Doctor Sabbatical spoke gently with words that did nothing to calm the caution in the air. I wished I had asked more questions, but she left after a few more sentences of support and leaving me alone gazing at a drawn blue curtain to contemplate my existence.

The world spun slower after that conversation and all the pain and sickness in my body seemed to pause for breath. The gravity of my predicament had me now digesting my ciphered warning to 'prepare myself' and what the vague subtext meant. They say that in moments before you are going to die that your life flashes before you in a time lapse. I cannot say this was the case for me (as I was only thinking I might be about to die) but all that consumed me was an overwhelming sense of calm. No panic or stress, if this was going to be my time then so be it, twenty-nine was not a bad innings and on the plus side I had seen England lift the rugby world cup. In that room surrounded by blue curtains my brain swelled with possible outcomes and thoughts of loved ones. Unpacking my morality was a steady process which went on for about an hour when an Orthopaedic Doctor who had seen me before entered my temple. "We think the infection is in your back" he began to which I injected "because of the surgery," "right" he replied. Doctor Familiar was a nice guy who always told you everything straight. I admired that about him, and he spoke and moved as if time slowed for him even though he must have been extremely busy. It was now after midnight and the day needed to be closed off. Part of me wanted to ask all the big questions but there would be time for that and without a scan of my spine, nothing was set in stone. The Doctor explained I would be going back to the ward where I had been living previously. Round and round we go, but if coming back was to be, familiar surroundings always add comfort. Luckily my girlfriend had pre-empted this move and packed me a small bag with some comfortable sportswear. Whilst the hospital clothing range is infamous, it is not particularly dashing but does have a very useful button and clip system on the front for removing clothing with sensational vigour. The interaction with Familiar was over and a couple of hours later I was taken up to my old home by a hospital porter. For what should have been a dramatic moment, time seemed to jog round my body, much like a Hollywood movie with the protagonist heading into the final battle I felt prepared due to my recent memiors. As I rolled on by the nurse's bay, Rachel, the nurse on duty at 3am remarked loudly "what on earth are you doing back here?" which greeted me like an enormous olive branch. "Missed the food" I replied, to which we both laughed. I was shown to my new digs, which was in a different room and by a window and in the corner. All my roomies were asleep as I lay staring at the ceiling imagining if this move would be permanent or my last journey anywhere. Death didn't scare me which sounds ridiculous, but this was the last mirage of mind as my eyelids closed the proceedings on a very eventful day.

Same Old Thing

"Help me. Please Help me. Help. Can anyone hear me? Help me, please. Help me" was the noise that woke me up on my first morning back in hospital. "Can someone help me?" an elderly voice continued to echo variations in requests for help over and over again. "Please help me, I am dying" the din went on until a healthcare assistant arrived and asked, "What is wrong Arthur?" "Nothing" The old man replied in a snap. This seemed to annoy the man who had come to his aid, but this scenario confused me. Why had this man been asking for help with such determination and then when his wish was granted, reject it? This thought process was interrupted by Arthur starting his vocal practice once more "Please help me, can anyone hear me? Help me. For God's sake I am dying here!" This went on, for quite a while and when the same attendant returned to his bed side and enquired to what his problem was? "Nice cup of tea?" said Arthur "You have a cup of tea Arthur; it is there on your tray" came the answer which was far from satisfactory. "Don't like that, nice cup of tea and two sugars" Arthur begged. The young man nodded and took his leave as it dawned on me that this one-sided conversation would be a regular feature in my stay here. On the bright side, I had got through my first night without anyone smoking indoors so we will take that as a small victory.

The room that I was now staying in was one down from my usual hang out. Six beds again, with the upper right corner being my patch. All six beds were occupied, with Arthur opposite my corner without a window. The average age in the room was well over seventy with the man in the first bed on the left by the door in deep discussion with what looked like some consultants (you can tell this by the smart clothes they wear, very expensive look.) "We have been looking at your paperwork and we have noticed a DNR (do not resuscitate) notation" Mr Consultant informed a man in his seventies who was in the company of his daughter who was sat by her father's bedside. "I have been looking at your records and I see when you were with us last time you had some major work done on your heart" the consultant continued. "That's right, he came through that well" his daughter interjected, "he did, and in comparison this shoulder repair is a much simpler operation which is why we would like to check if you still wanted the DNR to apply?" the consultant asked to a blank faced Bill. Having a DNR means that if anytime during your operation where you are asleep and your heart stops then the instructions to the surgeons are to not make it beat again. We all remember George Clooney waving two electric paddles together and screaming "clear" before shocking the patient in an attempt to restore the heart, a DNR removes this drama or if you look at it plainly it lets you die by leaving your heart still and frozen in your chest. Naturally the daughter launched in "this is nothing like the heart thing Dad, can we take that off, things are much better now." Bill's silent response deafened the room. Picking up on the vibe the consultant took their cue to leave the family discussion "we will come back in little while" and popped out of the drawn curtains leaving the father and daughter alone. What followed was a man revealing that he had no intention of changing his DNR request and felt very strongly about it. "I have had many good years and seen you grow into a beautiful woman. Your late mother would understand but it is unnatural my love, if I have to go, then so be it." Bill spoke with the affirmation of a man who had made up his mind and if he was compos mentos, it was still his call. What followed was a reveal of how bad the heart condition had been, presumably he signed the DNR because if things had gone wrong in that state, he would not have had a good quality of life. Bill had survived that, and his daughter implored him to see that this shoulder operation was much simpler. Was it riskier because of his age and repaired heart? To Bill it mattered not as he ignored his daughter's wishes and she left our room very upset. This early exchange reminded me quickly of the fishbowl I had been thrown back into, a place where life and death are discussed as if asking "fancy a cuppa?" in your kitchen at home. You never quite get used to listening to these conversations but as ever the blue shields offered no privacy by being drawn.

Morning rounds were led by Rachel as she handed over to the day team of nurses and healthcare assistants. After my operation I had made the choice to have my head shaved, don't have any reason why but just felt like doing something radical in my control. Those who identified the ward alumni poked remarks such as "where's it all gone?" and "I almost didn't recognise you!" Familiar faces comforted me in a reality that coming back so soon after my surgery was not good news. The school reunion departed and the tea trolley rattled in with high hopes of my old mate Oli however a new face appeared offering a hot beverage. Thinking that Arthur would now cease his chance to get that elusive cup of tea the lady asked him "would you like a hot drink?" The response to which was silence as it seemed Arthur had gone back to sleep but no matter, the tea round would come again at eleven. After my big reveal at handover, a couple of old friends slipped in and said a quick hello. These exchanges were extremely touching and although ill health again clouded my sky, a spritely hello from the ward staff filled my heart with joy. You are under no illusion how many people must come and go through these doors so to be welcomed was warming. Talking to one of the sisters I was intrigued to find out if any of my old roomies were still inside or where they had ended up? Two had stayed after me and they were Gerry (the man with the glamourous wife) and Smokey (sure you remember him.) Gerry had been here until a week ago because of complications with his healing process after the operation, this was largely down to his age accordingly, but he could not get stable enough to walk and hence the physio team would not sign him off. He had left our room and moved to another but accordingly often popped back with his wife to see everyone and handed out baked goods. The stay in total for Gerry was nine and a half weeks living in hospital when he was only supposed to be in for a week of post-operative recovery. That sounded like a slog but knowing his upbeat character and with the strength of his wife, I am sure he endured. That brings me nicely on to a slightly more colourful acquaintance. Smokey had been moved also, to a ward where you are supposed to be closer to moving out of hospital, but the sister informed me his 'unique' behaviour continued. The council had not been hasty in securing housing, so the hospital was his home for a long time. He continued to break the rules but managed to allude being caught until one day he went for a stroll. The sister told me he had disappeared from his bed when accordingly informing the nurse on duty "just popping for a cig love" as he wheeled outside. During the time he was missing one of the physio team came to the sister with a photograph. Around a two-mile walk from the hospital was a MacDonald's restaurant. A leisurely walk for most but a man with a broken ankle in a cast and who was on bed rest orders it was far from the one. The image had Smokey red handed about a hundred yards from the fast food delights. When he returned to the ward and was questioned on his absence his response was "I was just sitting outside enjoying the fresh air." This was the last lie he would tell; the evidence was presented, and the game was up and his marching orders were given for deliberately lying and deceiving the team. I asked, "where did he leave to?" and the sister did not know any further details, you have to give it to the man, he is nothing but not resourceful. He had stayed in hospital for a total of seven weeks drinking, smoking inside and enjoying 3 square meals a day. I wondered where he was now with part of me knowing that he was not a bad person at heart, Smokey was his own man finding his own way. The ward could not get him out without a smoking gun and the photo proving he had walked two miles was more than enough ammunition. A man of little learning had found a loophole in the system, misbehave but keep it subtle and you can get away with murder. It is also worth noting at this point, the complaint I logged on the night he smoked a cigarette inside our ward has still not been received and it is well over the response time.

Conversing with the Sister was interrupted by another familiar voice erupting like a volcano. "Help me, please, is anybody there? Help me, I am dying" Arthur barked into the room. "How long has he been in here?" I asked the sister, "about two weeks, he is very confused and when he is not sleeping, he is screaming for help which he won't let any of us give him" she replied. Later, I would discover he refused to let anyone take blood from his arm convinced they were attacking him with weapons, which was causing serious issues as they needed to do certainly pathology tests. Being unhealthy in body is one thing but to be ill of mind is another. Listening to Arthur broke my heart because in his world his behaviour was normal and maybe all he really wanted was a nice cup of tea? The sister stood up and told me that a doctor would be along for an update of how I was doing. In a strange way, being on the ward with everyone was comforting in an odd manner. The madness calmed me as I sipped on a truly terrible coffee listening to a confused old man scream out for assistance. Home is where the ward is, for now anyway.

Tested

The temperature was down but the headache was kicking my ass. By now I had been loaded with antibiotics, fluids and painkillers which had certainly improved me from life ending thoughts on a kitchen floor. A little after nine on the first morning the blue curtains which framed my bed were pulled back and two orthoepic doctors entered, neither of which I recognised. One of the Doctors did all the talking whilst the other, which seemed more junior (based entirely on age) held a clipboard and looked on attentively. "You are going to have an MRI of your entire spine this afternoon, this will show us if there is an infection in your spine from the surgery. We have also contacted Mr Quiet that you are here and having these tests" Doctor New explained. They were not messing about which only indicated to me they thought this was serious. I had only ever had a portion of my spine scanned before (Lumbar region) but to have all of it would be lengthy and showed they were taking no risks. They also had another running theory but that would not be revealed until much later. "My headache is still pounding" I replied knowing this would be a good chance to get a doctor's advice on treating it as they have to sign everything off. "I have written you up for codeine, paracetamol, ibuprofen and morphine, which I am hoping will help" came the response. All those weeks of suffering with drug withdrawal for nothing, I was back on all the things that had sent my body into crisis mode and yet my heart did not careless. Doctor new finished with "any more questions?" to which I shook my head and was left to lie on my back staring at the ceiling. "You need to prepare yourself" spiralled across my thoughts like a malfunctioning firework. My Dad was on his way to visit me and whether or not to be transparent was troubling me. He didn't deserve any more bad news but lying to the man who had given me a new spine was not great. The drugs were working and despite my coffee I drifted off to sleep quickly.

I was woken up by a woman who was there to take my blood. This would continue every day I was in hospital as they monitored me closely. Not long after my family arrived and doing my best routine of being uplifted, I was desperate to tell them all I wanted was to give up. Seeing them raised my spirits a little but exhausted me as I refused to let on how bad things were. Lying to ones we love is explained beautifully at the climax of *Miracle on 34th Street:* "What's better? A lie that gives a smile or a truth that draws a tear?" They are talking about the existence of Santa, but it is still poignant. Nothing had been proven so there was no need to shout it from the roof tops. They hugged me and left me alone to ponder if my actions were selfish or stupid and even now the answer evades me. The solemn soliloquy was interpreted by a nurse coming in to tell me the hospital porter was here to wheel me down to imaging and off I went to get me back scanned, this time for free.

The waiting room for the MRI scan had me and a man on bed who looked extremely pale and out of sync. A very pleasant woman informed me there was a person being scanned at the moment and I would be next or the one after the next one. Confusion over why my place in the queue was up for debate was answered ten minutes later as I overheard a phone call being made. "We have Mr Jones with us and we see he had an operation on his head removing something. Would you be able to inform us if this was metal or if any fragments could possibly be in his head still?" The reason the imaging woman was so keen to ask this is because the MRI machine is a massive magnet. If you have any metal in your body, it will move when the scanner is turned on and if something is moving through your brain that could be quite bum out. "Can't we just risk it? Mr Jones asked. "We don't risk things here Mr Jones when it comes to your health" was the answer to his silly question. Suddenly images of brain flying out of Mr Jones head sprung into thought which would be well placed in a Quinton Tarantino film. The phone rang and the answer was this was a no go, bad for Jones but very good for me. Into the scanner I descended as it took over seventy minutes to complete the scan.

Back to the ward of dreams and Bill's bed was empty but still had his personal effects so he must have been in theatre. Arthur was fast asleep and the bed in the middle on the right next to mine was being stripped for its next customer. A healthcare assistant wandered over and as he took my observations, we began talking of what it was like to work here. "It is a great team, a real family. My wife is a sister here and it works well but we are hugely under resourced. This job is getting harder and with not enough people to help with the workload we are rushed off our feet" he shared. This was not a surprise, but it was alarming what he went on to share. "Take last week, we had a very volatile patient here who was unhappy being in the hospital and an alcoholic. One morning he called for the sister's attention and when she was bedside, he stood up and punched her square in the jaw knocking her off her feet" the man told me. "She was back in work the next day though." Listening to this was extremely difficult. The people who work in these hospitals are on the frontline with some of society's most vulnerable people. When I was in the private hospital you did not see this part of society simply because they cannot afford it and there is something backwards about that. The state serves us all and gets literally punched in the face for it. I would witness more of the staff's resilience on my third morning in hospital. When we rose on and the healthcare assistants were doing the morning observations. During this they discovered Arthur had been sitting in his own excrement for most of the night without telling anyone. Realising they needed to clean this up urgently they attempted to move Arthur so they could wash him down and change the bedding. All hell broke loose and I could hear arms flailing with screams of "Get off me, you're hurting me" being repeated loudly. They could not leave Arthur in this mess, so they continued, no doubt being hit and pushed several times. The bed change was done, and silence fell kindly on the room with the smell in the air not so pleasurable. The two members of staff who had cleaned up were one male and one female, both of whom were healthcare assistants. Fast forward a little later and the night staff have switched to the day team. One of the sisters finds herself next to Arthur who is very agitated and erupts in confession "the man who changed my bed choked me by the neck. He hit me over and over. He has to go." The sister was having none of it, but to think these people are cleaning faeces up and are physically roughed up as they do so are also accused of foul play shows the dark reality of the job. Not every patient is like this but these experiences made me even more aware how important it was to be as polite and kind to those that take care of you inside the hospital and put into context when I had grumbled in my office performing menial HR tasks. We really don't know how good we have it.

The MRI showed that there was some liquid which had leaked around where Mr Quiet had cut into my back. This was normal accordingly, but they still had a few more tests to perform. Doctor Familiar informed me they were also passing me onto the medical team. They would be looking in more detail where the infection was coming from as for now it seemed that the surgery was not the root of my sickness. I got the feeling this was a win for the Orthopaedic team as an infection caused by surgery was preached at a low percentage and nobody wanted those statistics to their name. Mr Quiet was accordingly still being updated but by day three had not visited me despite being in the building. Doctor Familiar noticed that I was disinterested in this conversation despite being given seemingly good news "is everything ok Craig, you don't seem yourself?" He was right in his assessment because I would have preferred to be told that there was an infection in my spine rather than not. The reason being it meant they knew the issue and had a plan. With the current state of play, my head pounded, and the world was becoming less interesting to be in each day. "Fine mate, just the head" came my answer and he took his exit. More questions, more headaches and more drugs. This was all consuming me like a blanket over a flame.

Doctor Medical made his entrance wearing a particular flare shirt later that afternoon. He explained that because my symptoms could be risen from more than my surgery, they would need to do the following tests:

1. CT Scan – Image of my brain to check for anything rogue. Luckily for me it does not show character flaws and poor tastes.

2. Ultrasound Scan – Image of my stomach, like teen mum except I am almost thirty and not expecting to give birth but with all the MTV drama.

3. Extensive Blood Tests – The pathology laboratory at this hospital could not test for rare and tropical diseases. So, my samples would be transported to a nearby facility where they go full Pinky and the Brain.

4. Chest X-ray – Again, but hey, better safe than sorry?

This would give the medical doctors a full picture of what was going on in all aspects of my body and hopefully how to treat what was causing my symptoms. Doctor Medical spoke with an interest that connected me. Since arriving in A & E the orthoepic team seemed very panicked that the operation had caused my sickness which could involve a scolding because sloppy work and you must see teacher. This did nothing to reassure me of what was going on inside my body. The way they are looking at it is to save your life because if my back operation had caused Sepsis and this travelled to my major organs via transport of my blood then my curtain call was nearing. Doctor Medical asked me in detail about my headache and offered empathy on how crap my recent circumstances had been. Admitting that I thought it was all in my head was not easy but he reassured me this was normal. "Asking for help when things go badly is very difficult. Most people I meet have only come to hospital when the body is in it's worst condition" he shared. He was right, certainly about us British because we have to 'Keep Calm and Carry On' even if you have a lump on your arm or blood in your urine. Being in pain or having strange things happening in your body is one thing, but admitting you are sick and accepting the slog that comes after is fucking tough. If time travel was possible, I would have gone straight to a doctor the minute the leg twitched with pain in June 2018, hind sight is for mugs and makes us over think far too much. The good doctor was finished and implored me to hang tight as they would figure this all out which in that moment my heart believed, even if my head didn't.

That evening Rachel was back on night shift and someone had called in sick which meant they were a team member down with ten minutes notice. Seemed strange that nurses can pull a sicky but they are human after all. This put a huge amount of stress on the night staff which was noticed by those in my room. My new neighbour was an opinionated man who had a lot to say. "I need my medicine at 8pm and it's now 9pm, where the hell are you?" he bellowed into the corridor. Rachel eventually came by at half nine and administered our drugs apologising profusely as she did. Mr Opinion went fully in on her and I was furious. Rachel was a wonderful nurse who worked hard, was kind and a treasure to be in the company off. She was busting a gut to keep the ship sailing and this guy was giving her grief. Rachel just smiled in the face of adversity and went about her job with total professionalism. Be more like Rachel and the world would be a better place.

After seeing the shouting match at the nurses and listening to Arthur begin screaming again, I needed some peace and quiet so took myself off for a walk. It was sometime after ten and dark outside. The busy corridors which are crowded in the day were peaceful and still. Not even a mouse stirred in these aisles of half-light. The last two visits to hospital had left me unable to walk so this moment of exploration was a new one. Channelling thoughts of my mother and all the hours she had spent living in a hospital I found myself at the chapel. A small room with a dozen wooden pews filled the room with a stained-glass window of rainbow colours in the corner. Two solitary candles burned on a table at the front as I took my place on the third row and opened my mind. Raised as a Methodist was a stretch, but my secondary school had us in chapel twice a week and learned in classic hymns such as *Shine Jesus Shine*. God is not someone Craig knows but being here gave me some peace. Thoughts turned to my late mother and where she was right now. I yearned for a sign or some maternal wisdom to give me strength, but nothing happened and that was fine. Sitting still and taking stock of my recent months events I was filled with no emotion but just viewed the memories clearly. Sulking is not the answer when things get difficult and even if your life is at risk, better to rage against the end and not go gently into that good night. Mum had been in a hospital and when leaving she was told six weeks of her life remained. The time she actually had was two days. Seeing her trying to breathe and turning blue before death showed her strength and bravery. Even as her body failed her, my mother's spirit raged like a fantastic bonfire. She was a perfect example of never giving up and yet here her son was throwing in the towel after a bad few months. I am my mother's son and in that moment in a cramped chapel in an NHS hospital I was done with feeling sorry for myself because Que Sera Sera. I am not saying that we should compare ourselves to people dying and this will provide you with the perspective to complete life but if you have it in your arsenal it cannot hurt. In that moment I needed to be outside my thoughts, and I should have done this much sooner. For whatever reason life got easier in that moment because for now I was alive. Getting up slowly and whispering words of love to the heavens meant for my mother ended my divine intervention. I drifted back to the ward with watery eyes and got into bed with my mind buzzing. "Can somebody please help?" rung out in the room and after the third utterance I got up and walked out. Arriving at the nurse's station I told the Night Nurse "I think Arthur needs some help" and with that my day was to end.

Sitting, Waiting, Wishing

On the morning of my fifth day in hospital the arrival of Mr Quiet had everyone's attention. "I can now inform you that the infection has nothing to do with your spine or surgery and we also have eliminated the possibility of you having meningitis" were his opening remarks. Hang on a second, "What do you mean meningitis?" I asked with genuine intrigue as this had been the first mention of a pretty scary word. "One of the main theories for your symptoms was meningitis and that is all clear now so you can go home" Mr Quiet announced confidently as he now had scientific proof that this problem was not born of his handywork. "I haven't had any of the tests that the medical doctor had asked for. I was assuming those were taking place today" I asked a deflating Quiet. Unsure of what to answer or unbothered as this was not his area he turned to his accomplish who confirmed I was booked in for these tests later that day. "They will be in charge from here" he added before asking me to show him my back. Like Cristiano Ronaldo jumping up and landing in a power stance after scoring a prolific goal, Mr Quiet admired his craft with a plethora of language which stroked his ego with arrogance that was irritating. In a flourish he was away like a death eater with better places to be leaving me to ponder another thrilling engagement.

Now we know what 'prepare yourself' meant, they thought I might have bloody meningitis. Certainly, dodged a bullet there as that could of iced my cake which would have carried me over the sea of souls and right into Hades' front door. Having Mr Quiet appear after it was

159

proven that his work was all kosher angered me. The man had been in the same building since my day of arrival which made me think he was maybe biding him time to arrive with good news only. Infection chances from my operation were minimal and for a man that does hundreds of operations a year, bad stats can't be awesome for business. By this point my mind had arrived at the conclusion it didn't like Mr Quiet because he was intimidating, arrogant and unlikable. This may have been harsh as he had fixed my spine, but honesty is the best policy and he is one of the least likeable people in this story.

Busy day of tests ahead and my first interaction was an uplifting one. Spine clear and for the first morning inside the hospital I felt better. No sign of Oli the tea lad, which made me think maybe he had moved on in the world. Mid-morning had me down at the CT machine having a scan of my brain which was all clear and took all of an hour there and back. The afternoon had me playing a pregnant mum in EastEnders as they lubed up my stomach for an Ultrasound. "Is it a boy or a girl?" did not get a laugh from the woman performing the scan but made the nurse chuckle. "Everything looks clear" said the lady who had scanned me and afterwards a nurse wheeled me outside to wait in a long queue of patients who needed to be portered back to the wards. Being in a wheelchair I took stock of my surroundings in the imaging department of the hospital. This would be a place that would bring the best and worse news to all of those that enter. An MRI had solved the mystery of my spine but not given any clues as to what had caused me to be so sick again. A man was wheeled dramatically through the main doors with a bang wearing a blood-soaked head bandage dressed in clothes stained with a rich red shape. He looked in pretty bad shape as he was moved quickly into a room, "must have banged his head" I thought as he vanished out of sight. Nearly everywhere you go in this hospital is busy. Staff jog or run whilst waiting rooms swell over capacity. Something has to break soon in this fragile pyramid of cards but once you're inside it, you cannot stop but wonder at its magnificence. Organised chaos my old French teacher would label it. All that thinking must have worn my simple mind out because a kind hospital porter woke me up forty minutes later. Must have dosed off, just like on holiday, if you take your breaks in hospitals and feel crap throughout (may have just described a Benidorm hangover.) Gliding through the halls like Bambi on ice off the chair I got and into my corner bed. Both CT and Ultrasound were clear. How do you know that, you have not had a doctor tell you? Top Tip: You can ask the people that scan you if "everything looks ok?" From their response you get a quick answer:

- Nothing given away paired with "the doctor will be able to go into more detail" VERY BAD, you're probably going to die.

- "I am not sure but I will get someone who does" paired with a kind attitude, could be either way, less chance of RIP.

- Open and calm presence "All looks good Craig" and you're plain sailing.

Having put this scientific and surprisingly accurate test to use both times had confirmations of all clear which they would only do if you were. No one is going to confirm something without factual proof because no one wants a lawsuit on their head. Friday's flutters finished in a blossom of fish and chips on a plate which were surprisingly tasty. Mashing my peas onto some chip's thoughts drifted towards leaving. The headache was a 4/10 (back to NHS scale, much easier) and everything else was seemingly calming down. Leaving my bed after dinner to again exercise my right to corridor creep got my mind racing again. My destination was the canteen as a nurse had told me it stays open until about eight in the evening. Upon getting there, it was empty and being shut down but it was surprisingly impressive. One could get takeaway pizza, burgers and all sorts of cuisine to go. Missing serious tricks here, as I paid for a muller rice and took leave for the ward. The hospital felt like home by now as it understood what was going on and made me feel safe which I never really truly had at the private one. Thousands of people die here and the same amount get saved, the realities of these lives drip from the walls like sweat. The curiosity that was circling in my head must have been because the sickness was getting easier and I was getting better because when you feel terrible your brain focuses all its attention on pain rather than the diner's food menu. When back in bed I placed my headphones in and was able to watch a film without the volume feeling like a needle poking my brain over and over and over and over and over like a monkey with a miniature cymbal. Even resting becomes boring if you do enough and plans were brewing for me to get out and get my life back on track.

Saturday morning and I wake up full of beans. Headache is now a 3/10 and my body is feeling energetic for the first time, it was time for home. When the healthcare assistant came to give me my breakfast of cornflakes and one slice of cold toast, I asked to see the doctor on duty. Being a weekend, the hospital slows to a crawl as there are much fewer Doctors working covering a larger amount of patients. Smokey used to joke that the weekends were the best because you get away with anything you want, and he was right. Less staff equals less supervision ergo chaos reins down. Much to my surprise a young doctor came to my bedside within a few hours to assist me but today was not my day. "I have checked it out and given that your extensive blood tests have not been returned it is not safe for you to leave the hospital" came the response which was not the news we wanted. It was pointless asking how long the results would take as experience proved it would certainly not be until Monday. "Thank you for coming to see me so quickly" left my mouth as the doctor hurried onto his next patient. Frustration brewed in my loins, but we must listen to the experts even if every part of me wanted to walk out the front door. It is worth noting that hospital teaches you patience in abundance. Previous iterations of Craig would have told the doctor he was leaving and packed his bag and left which would have been stupid (and true to character.)

Later after lunch the healthcare assistant who had shared stories of how hard it was working here was by my bedside once again taking my blood pressure. "It is a good thing you are staying here until they finish the tests. We had a man a few weeks ago who came in with an unknown virus. One minute he was fine and talking and the next he turned grey and was taken to the ICU (Intensive Care Unit.) He passed away a few hours later, so it is good to take these things seriously." This man was not wrong and that shut me up about complaining. Things can change in a split second and being in a hospital, you are never going to go without care so safe is better than sorry, because if you are sorry, you're literally dead.

Bill was leaving our ward today and had made it through his shoulder surgery without any complications. His daughter beamed with sunshine as she helped her Dad pack up his things. Happy endings in these walls never get old and although I never spoke to them, I wished them a silent farewell as they left. Arthur had enjoyed a very busy morning in which they had finally be able to give him a bed wash properly. They brought a basin of hot soapy water and gently sponged his body clean. "That feels nice" he squealed as they wiped his legs. This was the first positive sentence I had heard come from his mouth in nearly a week and it made me smile. When the bathing was complete Arthur was like a cat who got the cream and asked his assistants as they left for one more request: "tasty bacon sandwich with butter and ketchup please." This had the whole room erupt into laughter and naturally we all started to joining in. "Whilst you're there, a cheeky Chinese will do me" one patient asked to which I added "domino's pizza for me, with lots of garlic and herb dip." The staff then added what they would like as if a takeaway bonanza was really possible. It was a beautiful moment that united patients and staff in unison, all human and all lovers of delicious food. The excitement clearly remained with Arthur as an hour later when playtime was over, he started to shout again "where is my bacon sandwich then?" which was certainly the biggest laugh of the day. Smiling felt marvellous that afternoon because we all felt part of something good and that is not a regular occurrence whilst in hospital.

Takeaway heaven was realised when my sister arrived on the Monday with a MacDonald's. Quarter pounder with cheese and a big old box of chicken nuggets was the literal one. Just before my sibling had arrived an orthopaedic doctor had come to visit me. "We have been told that you were asking to go home at the weekend?" This sounded like good news. "We have not had your blood results but given your mood and observations, discharging you today seems like a good idea." This was a massive win. My headache was a mild 2/10 and the big bad world was calling my name. This news was met with elation and praise from me as I launched into a speech thanking them for all their hard work. The running theory was that I had caught a common virus but because my immune system was so weak my body was not able to fight and hence made a real song and a dance out of it. This could have played out in a different way and they had done all they could to check me thoroughly. Whilst the discharge was being processed, I sat in the sunshine in the hospital garden chomping a burger with my sister. We chatted about nothing in particular but for the first time in a long time that was perfect. Conversations had been plagued by my persistent bad news but not today. My time in hospital was over for now and it all felt a little poetic. Later that afternoon I was wheeled to the front door by the same healthcare assistant who had shared so much with me "guess you are one of the lucky ones?" rung out as we headed to the main entrance. He was right but only because of those around me. My father once told me there is no such thing as luck, he defined it as "hard work coming into contact with opportunity." I would edit this for people in hospital to: hard work coming to contact with compassion and selfless efforts of hospital staff. There is no way I could be here writing this book without the help and care of so many unsung heroes. These people are in hospitals on Christmas day or in the middle of the night creating luck for vulnerable people and I do not know enough words to express my gratitude. I simply finished my scene by thanking him for wheeling me out and for everything to which he replied, "come and visit us soon, just not as a patient!" We both laughed and with that my lift home arrived and that was that, another level completed and back to normality I would go.

The Hill, The View and The Lights

July 1st 2019 was my last post-operative appointment at the private hospital with Mr Quiet. Using my new ability to walk with confidence (think Richard Ashcroft in the *Bittersweet Symphony* music video) I had made my way over via public transport which was a first. Using my legs with no pain in them felt amazing and as cheesy as it sounds, I wanted to rinse it. Sign into the front desk and my old friend the coffee machine made me an espresso (the diet had begun to transform me from fat slob back into slightly less chubby slob so mochas for now were having a small but not indefinite vacation.) Sitting in the familiar waiting room I took stock of my surrounds. I had entered this building many times being unable to walk, drugged up to my eyeballs and full of resentment. Having a pain free mind gifted me a clarity of thought of how far I had come. Hindsight is a wonderful thing but the last year had taken everything from me and this was a new start at the tired game of life. Plush chairs, snazzy decorations and a sense of calm sits in the air of the private hospital which in essence could not be more different to its NHS sibling. Gratitude was flowing through my heart followed by a trail of sadness, for not everyone is as lucky. My retrospective soliloquy was interpreted by a kind voice who beckoned me. I stood up and walked towards Mr Quiet's office for the last time.

"How are you feeling Craig?" was my greeting which caught me off guard. This seemed to be dressed in genuine concern. The ice was melting slowly in the kingdom of Narnia and my surgeon was growing a personality. Mr

Quiet then started explaining that all the checks had been very precise regarding my recent hospital visit and that he was happy to confirm nothing had gone wrong with the surgery. "It will take you around 3 months for the body to recover but your physio will go over this with you." A year after feeling a twitch in my left leg and I was finally on the real road to recovery. "I will remind you that running, and contact sports will be a long time away and please take any advice before engaging in such activities" came a final warning but that was fine. I could walk without pain, I could manage without medication and I felt back to my normal self with a hunger to make the most of my new lease of life. Maybe I had been too harsh on Mr Quiet, who is a fantastic surgeon (the neatness of my scar is testament to this) but lacks bedside manner. We shook hands and our friendship was over. Walking out of the private institution filled me with happiness because the worst was over, but part of my heart was heavy. How many people like Smokey, Gerry, Bill or Arthur could have prospered with these resources at their disposal? The NHS will fix you but unless your life is on the line you will wait for it. The time it took me to have my operation, be at home, have withdrawal and be back in hospital would be equal to the three month wait of my surgery on the NHS. I was extremely privileged to have a family that gifted me private healthcare but not everyone is so fortunate. Some politicians have argued that privatising aspects of the NHS is the answer to the funding crisis. This makes sense but it will leave the Smokey's of this world unable to access it. Our state funded healthcare set up is a blessing but one that is fragile. I don't know what the balance is, but money should not determine what care you receive. A recent study which The Guardian newspaper published revealed a terrifying truth: 'homeless people in England are 60 times more likely to visit A&E in a year." That means Smokey is statistically likely to come back into the hospital that he had been kicked out of. If graduate maths teachers are paid £26,000 in free bursaries to study a PGCE then student nurses should have their funding return. The NHS cannot continue as it is but with the current set up you can understand why a fundamental gap has emerged in healthcare students in this country. Save the nurses and save the world is what I believe but you have to go through it to fully understand. The only positive my operation gave to the NHS is a hope that someone else who was just as bad got their surgery a little quicker because I switched to the private sector. Mr Quiet informed me that his replacement had started in the NHS hospital I first met him at. "Are you retiring?" I asked before I left his flashy office. "Just from the public work, I am going to continue in the private sector a little longer" he replied. Guess he must be a fan of the free mocha's too.

The last year has been hell. The pain in my leg has been so bad I have been bed bound, unable to walk, sit, bend down or stretch and turn around. I was loaded on drugs that messed me up physically and mentally. Bitterness, pity and shame became my daily elixir of negative cocktails that inebriated my soul with a darkening shadow. I lost my job at a great company and almost lost the love of my life. I was depressed, suicidal and was void in all of life's wonders. I am not afraid to announce my bad experiences because it is imperative in me moving on.

Having spent a huge amount of time in the world of drama it seems fitting I close this tale with a Shakespearian reference, even though I can already hear my friends mocking me for it: When King Richard II is locked in a dungeon in Pomfret castle he contemplates his life shortly before he is murdered. This young king has abused his state and power and been overthrown by his cousin Bolingbroke. "I wasted time and now doth time waste me." Richard shares with the audience in a moment of clarity too late to halt is impending fate. The last twelve months have shown me that I do not want to find myself on death's door in the same conundrum as the young king. Richard is allowed this moment of hubris by Shakespeare to give him humanity, but it represents so much more. My life has not been lived to its full potential. My family have gifted me privilege, education and love that few people can dream of. No longer will I waste the gift of life. This sounds very Hollywood but what I mean by it is simple: none of the small stuff matters. When you are fighting for your life the job, the salary, the car, the house and the set of china you use at Christmas means fuck all. People are the point. Family, friends, love and kindness give this world a beat in a symphony of disorder. Say thank you, text that person that makes you laugh and let the passengers get off the train before you board because when the fat lady sings those are the gems that will lighten up your face. I promise you that this behaviour is infectious in a really good way, not the leaking spinal fluid meningitis way which is actually quite bad. The whole back saga has taught me to just be grateful, because apart from my own issues, I met some incredible people who showed me that life can be wonderful even in its final act.

In other news, I got a job. Only a temporary one but doing the beloved HR once more. Working in a college is great and I am surrounded by great people. The best bit about the role is that I can walk there, and this journey is giving my body a gentle piece of exercise as it rebuilds to the former glory of forgotten days. Being back in a professional environment was terrifying for the first few weeks as I was unsure if all the drugs and the drama had turned my brain into mush. It was a slow process but amazingly the work was possible and after a while I was even starting to enjoy it. My father always instilled me with the mantra 'feel the fear and do it anyway' (which is a self-help book, I think) and this could not have been truer. Trepidation is part of daily life and adds an edge or excitement to our activities. The difference now for me is that nothing is going to be as scary as being told to "prepare yourself to die" so everything must be a breeze now (I hope.) We are all on a journey up a hill of varying inclines, but we must remember to take a look around because the view is always there even if we fail to notice it.

Some people in this book are dead and whilst that is sad it is also life. Our time here is short, don't be a dick and waste it. Be the best you can be and do what makes you happy because we are all on borrowed time. Lastly, don't forget to smile because you might just surprise them.

Printed in Great
Britain
by Amazon

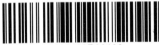